Dear Reader,

Changing what and how you eat can be a process. A lot of eating plans out there promise big results, but with a catch: You have to make big sacrifices too. It's true that changing your lifestyle requires you to change things you're doing daily, and sometimes that means forgoing a habit you've come to like. But life is meant to be enjoyed, and food is a **part of that enjoyment**.

Because I'm a nutritionist, you probably expect me to be one of those people telling you that you should be making healthy food choices—and sacrifices—*all* of the time, but I know just as much as anyone else that that's not realistic. I also understand that keto diets or cutting out carbs aren't the approaches that everyone wants to take. Thankfully, **there are other options**, and the macro diet is an excellent one.

The macro diet gives you more flexibility in your daily diet. While it's a good idea to make nutrient-rich food choices most of the time, this dietary plan lets you fit in your favorite foods while still hitting your goals. The bottom line is that with a macro diet, you make the rules. With a bit of nutrition and meal prepping guidance from me, you will get to decide **what works for you** and what doesn't. And once you realize you have the power to change your life, that's when the real magic happens.

Lindsay

Welcome to the Everything® Series!

These handy, accessible books give you all you need to tackle a difficult project, gain a new hobby, comprehend a fascinating topic, prepare for an exam, or even brush up on something you learned back in school but have since forgotten.

You can choose to read an Everything® book from cover to cover or just pick out the information you want from our four useful boxes: Questions, Facts, Alerts, and Essentials. We give you everything you need to know on the subject, but throw in a lot of fun stuff along the way too.

question

Answers to common questions.

fact

Important snippets of information.

alert

Urgent warnings.

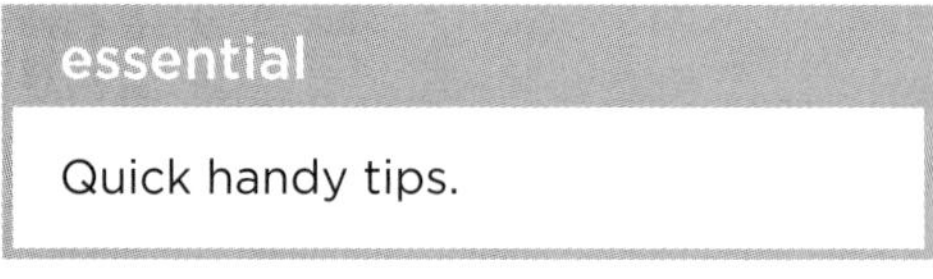

We now have more than 600 Everything® books in print, spanning such wide-ranging categories as cooking, health, parenting, personal finance, wedding planning, word puzzles, and so much more. When you're done reading them all, you can finally say you know Everything®!

PUBLISHER Karen Cooper

MANAGING EDITOR Lisa Laing

COPY CHIEF Casey Ebert

PRODUCTION EDITOR Jo-Anne Duhamel

ACQUISITIONS EDITOR Rebecca Tarr Thomas

DEVELOPMENT EDITOR Sarah Doughty

EVERYTHING® SERIES COVER DESIGNER Erin Alexander

THE EVERYTHING® MACRO DIET MEAL PREP COOKBOOK

LINDSAY BOYERS, CHNC

200 DELICIOUS RECIPES FOR A FLEXIBLE DIET THAT HELPS YOU LOSE WEIGHT AND IMPROVE YOUR HEALTH

ADAMS MEDIA

NEW YORK LONDON TORONTO SYDNEY NEW DELHI

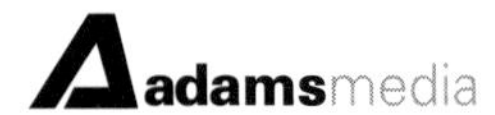

Adams Media
An Imprint of Simon & Schuster, Inc.
100 Technology Center Drive
Stoughton, Massachusetts 02072

An Everything® Series Book.

First Adams Media trade paperback edition March 2022

Interior layout by Alaya Howard
Photographs by James Stefiuk

Manufactured in the United States of America

1 2021

Library of Congress Cataloging-in-Publication Data has been applied for.

ISBN 978-1-5072-1813-6
ISBN 978-1-5072-1814-3 (ebook)

Contents

CHAPTER 9: SIDE DISHES 193

CHAPTER 10: SNACKS AND APPETIZERS 219

CHAPTER 11: SWEETS AND TREATS 243

Introduction

The macro diet is a powerful tool for your health that can reduce body fat, combat cravings, and help you reach your fitness goals. It may also help protect against diabetes and cardiovascular conditions. How? By focusing on counting macronutrients—carbohydrates, protein, and fat—in a more lenient way than the keto diet. It lets you enjoy a wide variety of your favorite foods without putting strict limits on any particular food group. It is also extremely customizable based on your goals. Want to lose weight? You can decide to cut carbs a little more. Want to build muscle? Ramp up your protein goals and make sure you're hitting them as closely as possible every day. No matter what health goals you have, the macro diet can help you get there.

And when you combine the macro diet with meal prepping, things get even simpler. While the macro diet gives you flexibility, meal prepping ensures that you always have a personally macro-balanced meal ready to eat any time you need it, so you don't fall off track. You can plan your days and even weeks in advance, batch cook, and then enjoy your meals with as little effort as possible. Prepping meals will also save you money, and help you avoid convenient temptations like fast food.

In *The Everything® Macro Diet Meal Prep Cookbook*, you'll find two hundred macro-friendly recipes created with meal prepping in mind. From out-of-the-box breakfast options like Spaghetti Squash Breakfast Bake and Cottage Cheese Muffins, to satisfying dinners like Buffalo Chicken Mac and Cheese and Gouda-Stuffed Pork Chops, to snacks like Pumpkin Oatmeal Bars and Cheesy Protein Popcorn to keep you full all day, there is something delicious for every meal. And with the macro diet, you won't have to give up dessert: Dig into a Ginger Triple Berry Crisp or Carrot Cake Bites without the guilt! Each recipe provides information on how to tailor ingredients to match your specific macro goals, as well as easy storing and reheating instructions. You'll also find a chapter on the essentials of macro dieting and meal prepping, from how to calculate and track your macros to grocery staples and proper storage. And don't forget to check out the Two-Week Meal Plan in the back of this book. You can follow along with each recipe, or swap in your favorites.

It may take a little time to adjust to counting your macros and prepping meals ahead of time, but together, the two strategies are a powerhouse for health. Meal prepping will guarantee your success in making the macro diet a simple part of your life!

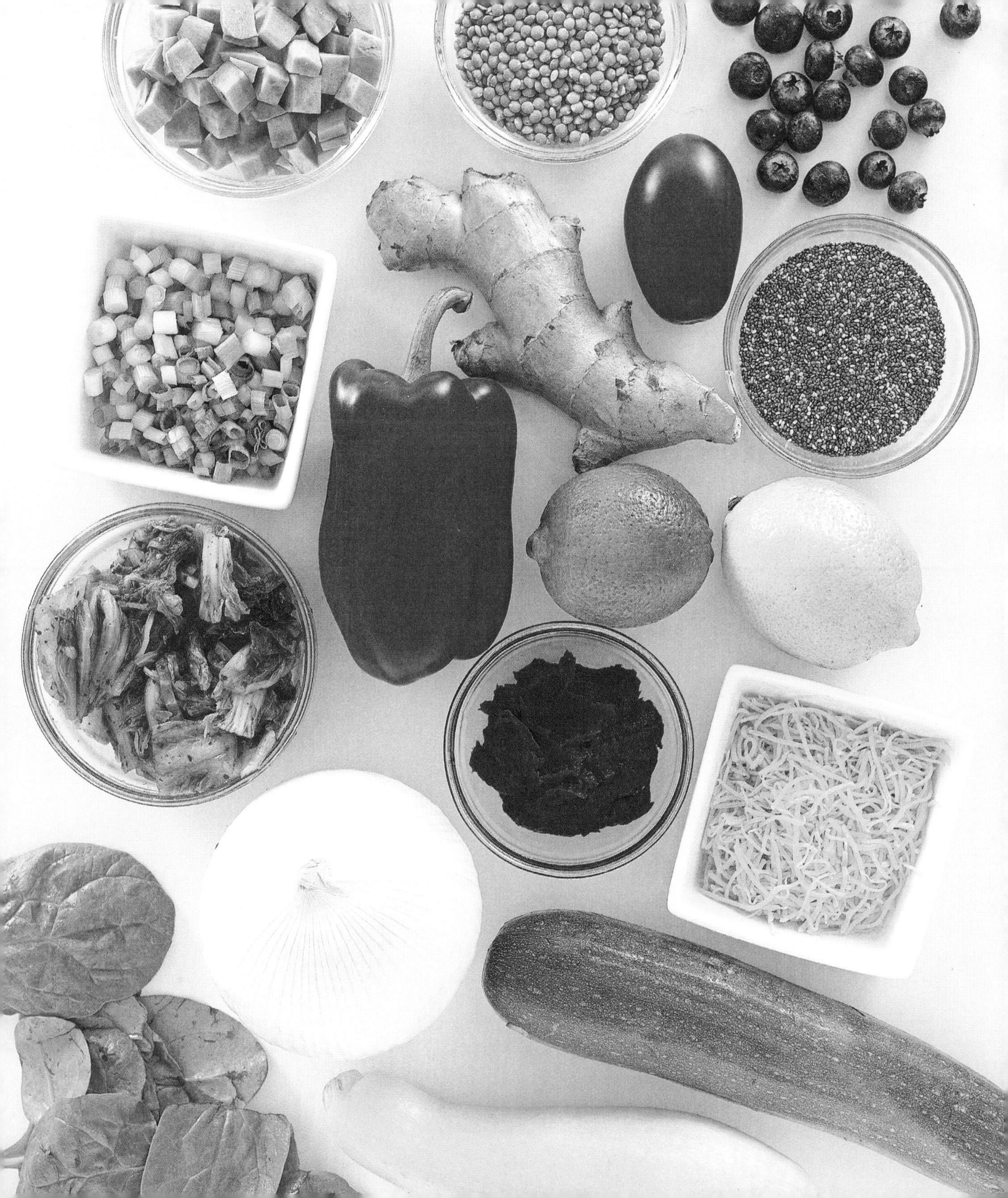

CHAPTER 1

Macro Diet and Meal Prep 101

When it comes to reaching your health goals, there are different recipes for success. What works for you may not work for your sister or best friend or co-worker. But because macro counting is so flexible, most people find enormous success with it. And when you combine it with meal prepping? It's almost impossible to go wrong. In this chapter, you'll explore the basics of the macro diet and prepping healthy meals, from how to calculate and track macronutrients to tips for successful meal prep.

What Is the Macro Diet?

The macro diet, often called "If It Fits Your Macros" or "IIFYM," isn't one specific diet but rather a set of principles that gives you a template for building out your meals. Instead of focusing on a set number of calories, the macro diet involves tracking your daily intake of macronutrients.

The Benefits of the Macro Diet

A properly balanced macro diet ensures that you're getting the right nutrition for your goals, whether that be weight loss, improved fitness, or just wanting to feel better, and that you're not over- or under-eating. This translates to better health and a reduced risk of chronic conditions, like heart disease, diabetes, and even Alzheimer's disease, down the road. A macro diet also allows more flexibility than other nutrition plans, since there are no strict food rules surrounding what you "can" and "can't" eat. You'll uncover more about the benefits of the macro diet and each macronutrient later in this chapter.

A Breakdown of Macronutrients

Before starting a macro diet, it's helpful to know what macros are and what they do for you. There are three macronutrients: carbohydrates, protein, and fat. Most foods contain some combination of all three, although there are foods that contain only one or two. For example, butter is mostly all fat with minuscule amounts of protein, while meat is mostly protein with some fat and zero carbohydrates. The calories in your food come from the macronutrients in that food:

- Carbohydrates have 4 calories per gram.
- Protein has 4 calories per gram.
- Fat has 9 calories per gram.

While calories are often described as some obscure measurement that pertains only to weight loss, they're actually units of energy. In other words, the calories in your food provide you with the energy you need to get through the day and perform basic, but necessary, functions like breathing and keeping your heart beating.

Some people say that it doesn't matter where your calories come from—that as long as you're sticking to your calorie numbers, you'll reach your goals. While that may be true in some ways, there's lots of science that says if you want to feel (and look) your best, it does matter where calories are coming from—and that's where the macro diet comes in.

Carbohydrates

The main function of carbohydrates, or "carbs" as they're often called, is to provide your body with energy. They exist in three main forms—sugars, starches, fibers—that can be further broken down into simple and complex carbohydrates.

You should prioritize complex carbohydrates over simple ones whenever possible.

Complex carbohydrates take longer to digest and thus provide a more sustained source of energy. Simple carbohydrates digest quickly and can provide an instant energy boost, but this is often followed by a crash that leaves you feeling hungry and worn out.

Complex carbohydrates are also often richer in fiber and starches, which have other health benefits. Fiber helps keep your digestion regular and can lower your risk of heart disease, while certain types of starches feed the good bacteria in your gut and help balance your gut microbiome.

> question
>
> **Which carbs are simple, and which are complex?**
>
> Simple carbohydrates are simple sugars that are found in foods like fruits, milk, and dairy products, as well as processed foods and drinks like white bread, candy, baked goods, and sodas. Complex carbohydrates are longer-chain sugars and starches that are found in foods like starchy vegetables, whole grains, and legumes.

Some of the best sources of carbohydrates in a macro diet are:

- Sweet potatoes
- White potatoes
- Brown rice
- Gluten-free rolled oats
- Legumes (beans, peas, lentils, chickpeas)
- Whole fruits
- Vegetables
- Nuts
- Seeds

Because carbohydrates are such a convenient source of energy, your body always prioritizes using them over fats and proteins. In some ways, this is a good thing. But if you're constantly overeating carbohydrates, or any of the other macronutrients, it can lead to weight gain. That's why tracking is important. (More on that later.)

Protein

Protein is often considered the most important macronutrient when following a macro diet. While the ultimate goal in this diet is to nail your numbers every time, protein is a good place to start if you're new to macros.

Proteins have more functions than either of the other macronutrients. They're involved in your metabolism, build and repair your body's tissues, and help maintain proper fluid and pH balance. Proteins also provide the structural framework for all of your cells.

All proteins are made up of amino acids, which are often called the building blocks of life. When you eat protein, your body breaks it down into individual amino acids and then uses those amino acids to rebuild the new proteins you need to carry out daily functions. There are twenty standard amino acids. Nine of them are categorized as essential, and eleven are nonessential. Essential amino acids are those that your body can't make. The essential part comes from the fact that you must include them in your diet, otherwise your body won't have access to them. On the other hand, your body can make nonessential amino acids. They're not less important than essential amino acids; it's just not as vital to include them in your diet since your body can make what it needs.

fact

Of the three macronutrients, carbohydrates is the only one that's classified as nonessential. Your body is physically capable of obtaining all of its energy from protein and fat. This is the basis of low-carb and keto diets; once you teach your body how to thrive on fat as an energy source, your need for carbohydrates can lessen.

Proteins are further broken down into complete and incomplete proteins. Complete proteins provide all of the essential amino acids, while incomplete proteins are missing some. When choosing your protein sources, it's best to fit in complete proteins whenever possible. You can also make a complete protein by eating complementary proteins—two incomplete proteins that each have the essential amino acids the other is missing—throughout the week. Some examples of complementary proteins are lentils and quinoa, rice and beans, and peanut butter and whole-grain bread.

essential

As a general rule, animal-based proteins, like meats and eggs, are complete proteins, whereas plant-based proteins, like beans and legumes, are incomplete proteins. There are some exceptions to this rule, though. For example, nutritional yeast is a complete protein.

Some of the best sources of protein in a macro diet are:

- Lean meats (beef, pork, lamb)
- Poultry (chicken, turkey)
- Seafood (fish, shellfish)
- Eggs
- Grass-fed dairy products
- Nuts
- Seeds
- Legumes (beans, peas, lentils, chickpeas)

The protein from complete protein sources, such as lean meat and poultry, is more bioavailable, meaning your body can digest and absorb it better than protein from other sources. That said, it is possible to get adequate protein solely from plant-based foods.

Fat

Fat may be the most misunderstood macronutrient of them all. In the 1990s, many health experts pointed the finger at this macronutrient, suggesting that it was the sole reason for weight gain and many other health problems, including heart disease. But, as it turns out, many of those initial theories were wrong, and science shows that fat is an essential part of a healthy diet. It's true that fat has more calories per gram than the other two macronutrients, but you'll reap big rewards when you work it into your diet in a strategic way.

Your body uses fat as a secondary fuel source, and it's a major storage form of energy in the body. Fat also helps you absorb fat-soluble vitamins, cushions and protects your organs, helps you regulate your body temperature, and supports cell growth. Adding fat to your meals also helps you feel satisfied instead of unfulfilled after eating.

alert

You may have heard people refer to unsaturated fat as "good" and saturated fat as "bad." This is another oversimplified nutrition philosophy. The effect that saturated fats have on your body depends on the overall nutrient content of the food and your overall diet quality. For example, there are studies that show that consuming full-fat dairy, which is rich in saturated fat, has no negative effect on heart disease risk. Rather than vilifying saturated fat, be mindful of your sources and consuming it as part of a healthy diet.

Just as with proteins, there are essential fatty acids, like omega-3s and omega-6s. Since your body can't make these types of fats, you have to get them from your diet to feel your best.

Some of the best sources of fat in a macro diet are:

- Fatty fish (salmon, mackerel, herring, sardines, albacore tuna)
- Nuts
- Seeds
- Grass-fed butter and healthy oils (avocado, olive, sesame)
- Avocado
- Olives
- Grass-fed meats

The recipes in this book capitalize on the benefits of these and other good sources of fat.

How to Calculate Your Macro Goals

Now that you know what macronutrients are and where you can find them, another important piece of the puzzle is learning how to calculate your macro goals and track how many you're eating. The first step in calculating your macros is figuring out how many calories you need each day. The easiest way to do this is to use a free online calculator. Just search "calorie calculator" online, and you'll be met with many options that will let you plug in your specifics, from your height and weight, to your fitness goals. Once you have that number, you'll use it to calculate the grams of each macronutrient. Thankfully, there are online calculators and apps that will do most of this work for you; just search "macronutrient calculator" and/or "macronutrient tracker" and you'll get a ton of results.

Since the macro diet is adaptable, there aren't perfect macronutrient ranges that work for everyone, but here is a good starting point that online calculators work from:

- Carbohydrates: 30–40 percent of daily calories
- Protein: 25–35 percent of daily calories
- Fat: 20–30 percent of daily calories

Many people prefer a low-carb approach to macro counting. If you started a macro diet and you're not seeing the results you want, or if you prefer to limit your carb intake, your macro breakdown should look more like this:

- Carbohydrates: 15–25 percent of daily calories
- Protein: 40–50 percent of daily calories
- Fat: 30–35 percent of daily calories

Figuring out your macronutrient sweet spot may take some time and adjusting as you go, but once you pick a plan, give it a couple weeks to see how you feel and then you can change things, if necessary.

How to Track Your Macros

Once you've figured out your ideal macronutrient ranges, or the place you want to start, the next step is tracking your macros. The best way to do this is with an app that easily lets you plug in everything you're eating. A good macro tracking app will break down all of the food you're eating into carbohydrates, protein, and fat and show you where you stand for the day—and how many grams of each you have left. MyFitnessPal, MyMacros+, and LoseIt! are all excellent options.

A Note about Micronutrients

While the macro diet is of course built around macros, micronutrients (vitamins and minerals) are equally important. Each vitamin and mineral has its own specific function, and many of them work synergistically, or together, to make you feel your best. Vitamins and minerals support growth and development, ensure your organs are healthy and functioning properly, help your body make new red blood cells, keep your bones strong, and keep your immune system functioning properly. Micronutrients, like vitamin D and vitamin B_{12}, also play a serious role in your mental health. The macro diet doesn't make specific recommendations around micronutrients, but if you're getting less than you need, you'll feel it—physically and mentally. That's why it's important to make nutrient-rich, healthy food choices as much as possible.

When following a macro diet, you don't have to track micronutrients (unless you want to). Instead, when you choose to fill your plate with vegetables, whole foods, and high-quality meats most of the time, you'll naturally hit many of your micronutrient goals as well. Granted, there will be some exceptions, especially for harder-to-get nutrients like vitamin D. This is where targeted supplements that are recommended specifically for you by a healthcare professional can come into play.

The Benefits of Meal Prepping

Once you've decided on your macro diet plan and how you'll track it, the next step is getting organized and setting yourself up for success, and you can do this through meal prepping. During meal prepping, or preparing dishes or meals in advance, you will set aside a few hours of time to batch cook meals for the week ahead. After you cook your meals, you will divide them into individual servings and store them until you're ready to eat.

Meal prepping certainly makes things more convenient, but the benefits extend far beyond that too. Research published in the *International Journal of Behavioral Nutrition and Physical Activity* shows that meal prepping can help improve your diet quality, contribute to eating more food variety, and help you maintain a healthier body weight.

Meal prepping also:

- Saves money
- Saves time, even though it may feel like more work in the beginning
- Reduces overall stress, particularly stress around food decisions or last-minute food preparation
- Reduces temptation and makes it less likely that you'll succumb to temptation
- Helps manage hunger, since you always have a macro-balanced meal at your fingertips
- Prevents overeating since meals are already portioned out
- Gives you total control over meal ingredients and what you're eating

Meal prepping helps take the macro diet to the next level.

Meal Prepping Tips

When it comes to meal prepping, organization is the key to success. Initially, it may seem like a lot of extra work—and a lot of time spent—but once you get the hang of it, you'll realize that you're actually saving both time and money. Many people choose to spend a few hours cooking on a Sunday to prepare meals for the entire week. Others do shorter cooking bursts a couple times a week. Whatever you decide to do, here are some tips that can help you out:

1. **Make Your Plan.** The first step is figuring out your meals and eating schedule. You can sit down on a Sunday and map out what you're going to eat for the week ahead, or make a month-long meal plan. Or you may decide to start

with just a few days and see how you fare. Regardless, you'll want to write down exactly what you'll be eating for each meal and snack.

2. **Set the Schedule.** Once you decide what you're going to eat, the next step is figuring out the execution. Are you going to set aside a few hours on the weekend to grocery shop and cook? Or are you going to plan a few days at a time and divide up the effort?
3. **Take Stock of Your Pantry.** Before writing your grocery list, figure out what ingredients you *don't* need. This way, you won't buy extras and have them go to waste.
4. **Write Out Your Grocery List.** Organize items by where they're found in the grocery store. Put all produce items together, canned items together, meats together, and so on. This way, you won't have to spend time backtracking when you're shopping or re-reading your list.

A well-thought-out plan and organized list will help ensure a smooth meal prepping experience.

Buy in Bulk

Another way to save time and money when meal prepping is to buy whatever you can in bulk. You'll likely be using many of the same ingredients repeatedly, especially once you find a great schedule of recipes that perfectly fits with your macros, so buy items in larger quantities and stock them in your pantry and freezer, if you have the extra space. You may want to invest in a membership at a wholesale club like Costco or BJ's. There are also online membership-only markets, like Thrive Market, where you can purchase food at a discount and have it delivered right to your door.

Getting Organized on Cooking Day

Once you've grocery shopped, the next step is batch cooking. Many people like to shop and cook on the same day to avoid the extra step of putting away any perishable groceries, but do what works best for you. Here are some tips to help set you up for success:

- **Start with a clean kitchen.** Cleaning your kitchen and clearing away any unnecessary clutter will open up the space you need for batch cooking, and do wonders for your stress level.
- **Gather all your kitchen tools.** Take out all the pots, pans, cutting boards, and kitchen appliances you'll need to get the job done. That way they'll be easily within reach so you don't have to go searching with chicken juice on your hands later.
- **Batch cook whatever you can.** Look through your recipes and total up any common ingredients. For example, if two recipes call for ½ cup of brown rice and another two call for 1 cup of cooked sweet potatoes, make a note to cook a total of 1 cup of brown rice and 2 cups of sweet potatoes and divide it up later. This applies to prep work too. If you need three chopped onions total, chop them all at once.

- **Multitask as much as possible.** Rather than going through each recipe from start to finish, do a few tasks at once, if you can. Start up a batch of rice, and while that's cooking, chop up vegetables or prepare your slow cooker recipes.
- **Account for marinating time.** Some recipes require you to marinate meats and let them sit for an hour or two before cooking. Make note of these recipes so you can plan accordingly.
- **Clean as you go.** Rather than using every pot and pan in your kitchen, quickly wipe out used skillets or saucepans and reuse them so you have less to clean up when you're done cooking. Transfer scraps and packaging to the trash as you cook too.

essential

A great strategy when cooking is to double up or even triple up on your recipes to create freezer meals that you can eat later. If a recipe makes six servings, double the recipe and make twelve. Store six in the refrigerator for the week, then portion out the remaining six and put them in the freezer. If you do this every time, you'll eventually have a freezer stocked full of meals so you don't have to cook as often.

It's also helpful to lay all your recipes out where you can see them so you can cross-reference and double-check ingredients and steps as you go.

Storage and Reheating

Proper storage and reheating are other important components of meal planning and prepping. When figuring out how you want to approach this, these are your two main goals:

1. Ensure the food lasts as long as possible in the refrigerator or freezer while still remaining safe to eat.
2. Reheat the food in a way that preserves quality so the food will actually taste good when it comes time to eat it.

Spending a little extra time dividing your meals into portions before storing them will save lots of time when you're ready to eat, since you'll just have to grab a container and reheat the food.

alert

Plastic is often a go-to for meal prep, but it has several downsides, even beyond its negative impact on the environment. Plastic is porous, so it absorbs strong food flavors and stains more easily than other materials. It's also recommended that you don't microwave your food in plastic. For these reasons, it's best to store your food in stainless steel or glass containers. Glass tends to keep cooked food fresher for longer. Most glass is also microwave-safe, and some is even oven-safe.

Once all of your meals are assembled for storage, label each container with a piece of tape. Write the date the food was made and which meal it's for—for example, "Monday breakfast." Once each container is labeled, stack them in the refrigerator in the order you're planning to eat them.

When it comes time to eat, proper reheating goes a long way toward maximizing the flavor and texture of your meals. The best way to retain moisture and flavor is to warm up food slowly. That means heating the food in a skillet on the stove over medium-low heat, or warming it up in the oven at a temperature of 250°F to 300°F. The air fryer is also an excellent way to reheat food, especially if you want it to regain some of its original crispiness.

Of course, the microwave works if you're on the go and don't have access to any other heating methods, or if you're in a rush. The same rules apply though: Turn the power level down to about 50 percent and heat your food in 30-second increments, making sure to stir as you go since microwaves are notorious for uneven heating.

Getting Started

Meal prepping for a macro diet is a learning process that you can adjust to fit into your lifestyle. The point is to simplify your routine so that following the diet feels enjoyable, not like a chore or a source of frustration. If you're able to develop a plan that helps you stick to your diet and allows you to have fun doing it, that's a win!

CHAPTER 2

Breakfast

Cinnamon Roll Overnight Oats

SERVES 6

Per Serving:

Calories	238
Fat	7g
Sodium	101mg
Carbohydrates	36g
Fiber	12g
Sugar	2g
Protein	8g

CAN YOU HEAT OVERNIGHT NIGHTS?

Overnight oats are meant to be eaten cold, right out of the refrigerator, but if you prefer warm oatmeal, you can heat them up in the microwave or dump them out into a pot and warm them on the stovetop. Just keep the heat low and add a little extra liquid until the oatmeal reaches your preferred consistency.

These Cinnamon Roll Overnight Oats require absolutely no cooking and can keep in your refrigerator for almost a week. Just shake up the ingredients, let sit, and enjoy hot or cold.

3 cups gluten-free rolled oats
¾ cup full-fat plain Greek yogurt
3 cups unsweetened vanilla almond milk
3 teaspoons ground cinnamon
6 teaspoons chia seeds
3 teaspoons vanilla extract
6 teaspoons ChocZero Maple-Flavored Syrup

1. Scoop ½ cup oats, 2 tablespoons yogurt, ½ cup almond milk, ½ teaspoon cinnamon, 1 teaspoon chia seeds, ½ teaspoon vanilla, and 1 teaspoon maple syrup into each of six pint-sized Mason jars or other airtight containers. Cover and shake vigorously.
2. Refrigerate at least 4 hours before eating, and up to 6 days. Serve cold.

Spaghetti Squash Breakfast Bake

Spaghetti squash is normally reserved for dinnertime, but thanks to its neutral flavor, it makes an excellent addition to breakfast. Plus, it adds a small amount of complex carbs that help keep your day macro-balanced.

SERVES 6

Per Serving:

Calories	301
Fat	20g
Sodium	583mg
Carbohydrates	13g
Fiber	3g
Sugar	6g
Protein	17g

6 cups cooked spaghetti squash

6 large eggs, lightly beaten

1 cup crumbled cooked pork sausage

1 cup no-sugar-added salsa

½ cup finely chopped green bell pepper

1 cup shredded Cheddar cheese

1. Preheat oven to 350°F.
2. Add all ingredients, except cheese, to an 8" × 8" baking dish and stir until thoroughly combined.
3. Top with cheese.
4. Bake 30 minutes or until eggs are set and cheese is slightly browned. Remove from oven and allow to cool 30 minutes.
5. Cut into six equal pieces and transfer each piece to a separate air-tight container. Cover and store in refrigerator until ready to eat, up to 1 week.
6. To serve, heat in microwave 2 minutes, or transfer to a baking dish and bake at 300°F 30 minutes.

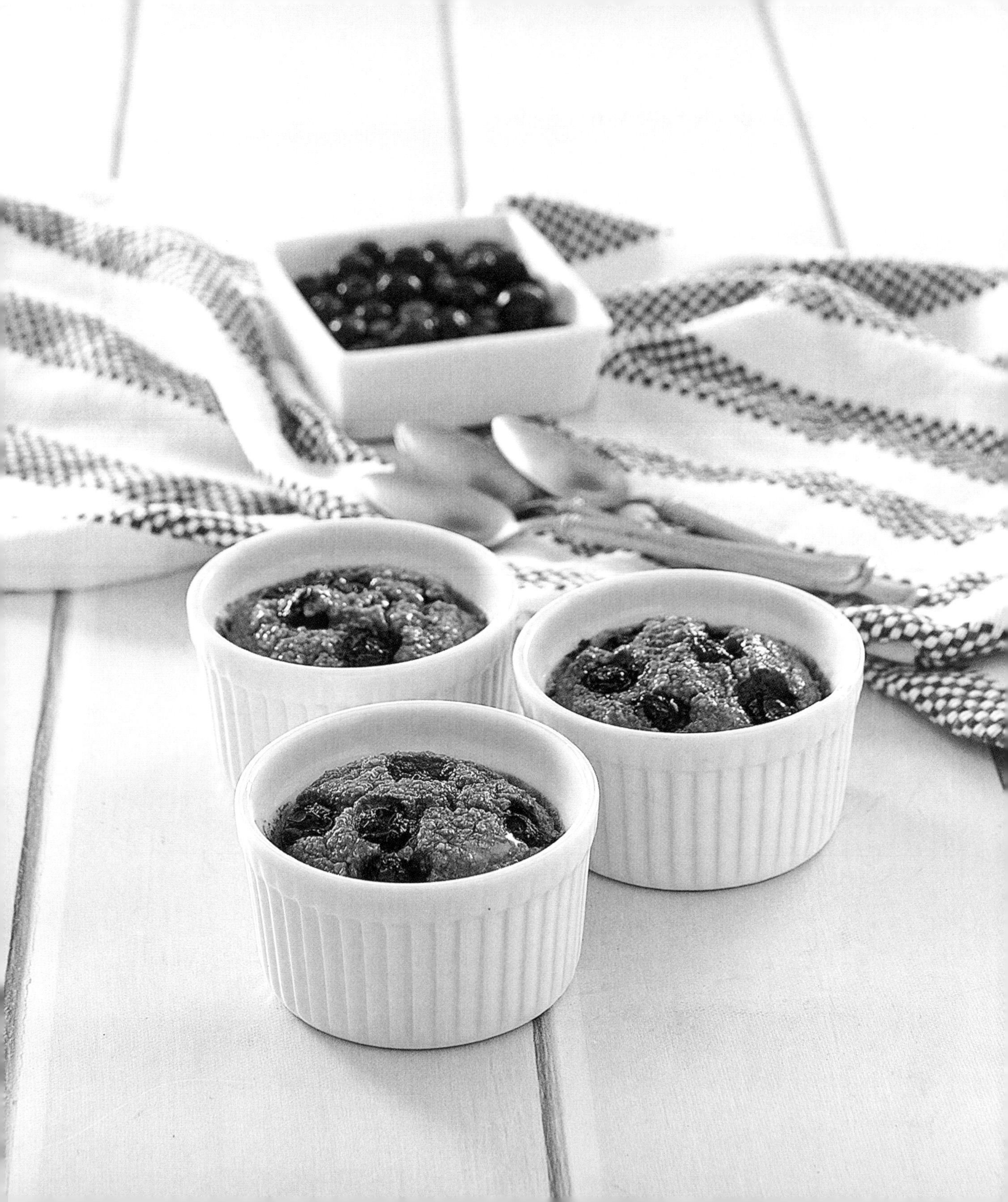

Blueberry Baked Oats

Baked oats are reminiscent of cake, but without any of the refined sugars. You can use any of your favorite fruit in place of the blueberries or switch things up by adding Lily's stevia-sweetened chocolate chips or chopped nuts in place of the fruit.

SERVES 6

Per Serving:

Calories	323
Fat	12g
Sodium	186mg
Carbohydrates	42g
Fiber	14g
Sugar	6g
Protein	12g

3 cups gluten-free rolled oats
½ cup unsweetened vanilla almond milk
2 small extra-ripe bananas
6 large eggs
3 tablespoons ChocZero Maple-Flavored Syrup
3 tablespoons no-sugar-added almond butter
1½ teaspoons baking powder
½ teaspoon ground cinnamon
¼ teaspoon sea salt
¾ cup frozen wild blueberries

1. Preheat oven to 350°F.
2. Add all ingredients, except blueberries, to a blender and blend until smooth, about 1 minute.
3. Stir in blueberries.
4. Pour equal amounts of batter into six 8-ounce ramekins. Place ramekins on a baking sheet and bake 25 minutes or until a toothpick inserted in center comes out clean. Remove from oven and allow to cool 1 hour.
5. Cover ramekins with plastic wrap and refrigerate until ready to eat, up to 1 week.
6. Serve cold, or heat in microwave 45 seconds or until just warmed through.

GO WILD

Any blueberries will work in this recipe, but wild blueberries are especially beneficial thanks to higher amounts of anthocyanin, the antioxidant that gives blueberries their characteristic color. Anthocyanins can help ward off heart disease, diabetes, cancer, and chronic inflammation. They can also help you maintain a healthy weight.

High-Protein Greek Yogurt Parfaits

SERVES 6

Per Serving:	
Calories	645
Fat	40g
Sodium	118mg
Carbohydrates	28g
Fiber	7g
Sugar	16g
Protein	44g

This recipe is easily customizable to your specific macros. You can use different types of yogurt (nonfat or reduced fat) if you need to cut back on fat or use an oat-based granola instead of a Paleo one for more carbs.

6 cups full-fat plain Greek yogurt

6 scoops Tera's Whey vanilla protein powder

2 cups frozen wild blueberries

¾ cup hemp hearts

2 cups Paleo granola

1. Combine yogurt and protein powder in a large bowl and stir until evenly incorporated.
2. Divide evenly into six pint-sized Mason jars. Top each with ⅓ cup frozen blueberries, 2 tablespoons hemp hearts, and ⅓ cup granola.
3. Cover and store in refrigerator until ready to eat, up to 1 week. Serve cold.

Chocolate Peanut Butter Chia Pudding Cups

SERVES 6

Per Serving:	
Calories	323
Fat	18g
Sodium	281mg
Carbohydrates	19g
Fiber	14g
Sugar	3g
Protein	23g

If you don't love the texture of chia seeds, you can make a smoother pudding by adding all the ingredients (except the chopped peanuts) to a blender and then dividing the mixture into six cups before letting it set in the refrigerator.

6 cups unsweetened vanilla almond milk

¾ cup chia seeds

6 scoops Tera's Whey chocolate protein powder

¾ cup powdered peanut butter

6 tablespoons chopped peanuts

1. Combine 1 cup almond milk, 2 tablespoons chia seeds, 1 scoop protein powder, and 2 tablespoons powdered peanut butter in each of six pint-sized Mason jars. Cover and shake each jar 30 seconds.
2. Stir 1 tablespoon peanuts into each jar, cover again, and let sit in refrigerator at least 4 hours or overnight. Serve cold.

Gluten-Free Protein Pancake Squares

This macro-friendly recipe is the perfect base for all your favorite pancake toppings. Instead of blueberries, you can use strawberries, bananas, chocolate chips, walnuts, or any mix-ins that fit into your plan. Eat the pancakes cold or heat them up for a minute in the microwave before enjoying.

SERVES 6

Per Serving:

Calories	366
Fat	15g
Sodium	752mg
Carbohydrates	31g
Fiber	13g
Sugar	4g
Protein	24g

2 cups Birch Benders Paleo Pancake and Waffle Mix

¼ teaspoon vanilla extract

1¾ cups egg whites

2 cups frozen wild blueberries

1. Preheat oven to 400°F.
2. Line a baking sheet with parchment paper and coat with avocado oil cooking spray.
3. Combine pancake mix, vanilla, and egg whites in a large bowl. Let sit 5 minutes, then stir in blueberries.
4. Spread batter evenly on prepared baking sheet and bake 10 minutes. Turn oven off and let sit in oven for 2 minutes or until batter is set. Remove from oven and allow to cool 30 minutes.
5. Cut into twelve squares. Store two squares in each of six reusable storage bags or airtight containers in refrigerator until ready to eat, up to 1 week.
6. Serve cold or heat in a skillet over medium-low heat 1 minute on each side.

Mexican Breakfast Bowls

SERVES 6

Per Serving:

Calories	413
Fat	22g
Sodium	698mg
Carbohydrates	30g
Fiber	4g
Sugar	1g
Protein	23g

MEAL PREPPING OVER-EASY EGGS

Hard-boiled eggs are typically the go-to for meal prep, but it's just as easy to prepare over-easy or sunny-side up eggs for the week. Instead of cooking them in a skillet, you can make a big batch in the oven. Heat your oven to 350°F, grease a baking sheet, crack 6–12 eggs on it (making the yolk as evenly spaced out as possible), and then bake for 12 minutes.

When meal prepping over-easy eggs, it's best to leave them slightly runny rather than overcooking them. That way, when it's time to reheat your meal, you'll end up with a perfectly cooked egg, rather than one that feels rubbery. Alternatively, you can prep just the sweet potato and chorizo mixture in advance and then cook your egg right before eating.

1 small yellow onion, peeled and diced

2 cups peeled diced sweet potatoes

1 tablespoon avocado oil

½ teaspoon sea salt

½ teaspoon ground black pepper

½ teaspoon chili powder

½ teaspoon ground cumin

1 pound ground chorizo

1 (15-ounce) can black beans, drained and rinsed

½ cup diced green bell pepper

6 large eggs

6 teaspoons Cholula Hot Sauce

1. Preheat oven to 400°F. Line a baking sheet with parchment paper.
2. Combine onion and sweet potatoes in a large mixing bowl. Drizzle with oil and toss to coat evenly. Sprinkle salt, black pepper, chili powder, and cumin on top and toss to coat.
3. Spread sweet potato mixture out evenly on prepared baking sheet. Bake 20 minutes or until potatoes are fork-tender, flipping potatoes once while cooking. Remove from oven and set aside.
4. Heat a large skillet over medium heat. Add chorizo and cook 2 minutes until fat starts to render, then add beans and bell pepper. Cook until chorizo is no longer pink and bell pepper is tender, about 7 minutes. Remove from heat. Drain chorizo fat into separate small bowl; set aside.
5. Fold sweet potato mixture into chorizo mixture, stirring carefully to combine. Divide mixture evenly into six airtight containers.
6. Reheat skillet with chorizo fat over medium heat. Add eggs and cook 2 minutes on each side. Place 1 egg in each container. Drizzle hot sauce on top.
7. Cover and store containers in refrigerator until ready to eat, up to 1 week. When ready to serve, heat in a skillet over medium-low heat 5 minutes, or microwave 1 minute, or until heated through.

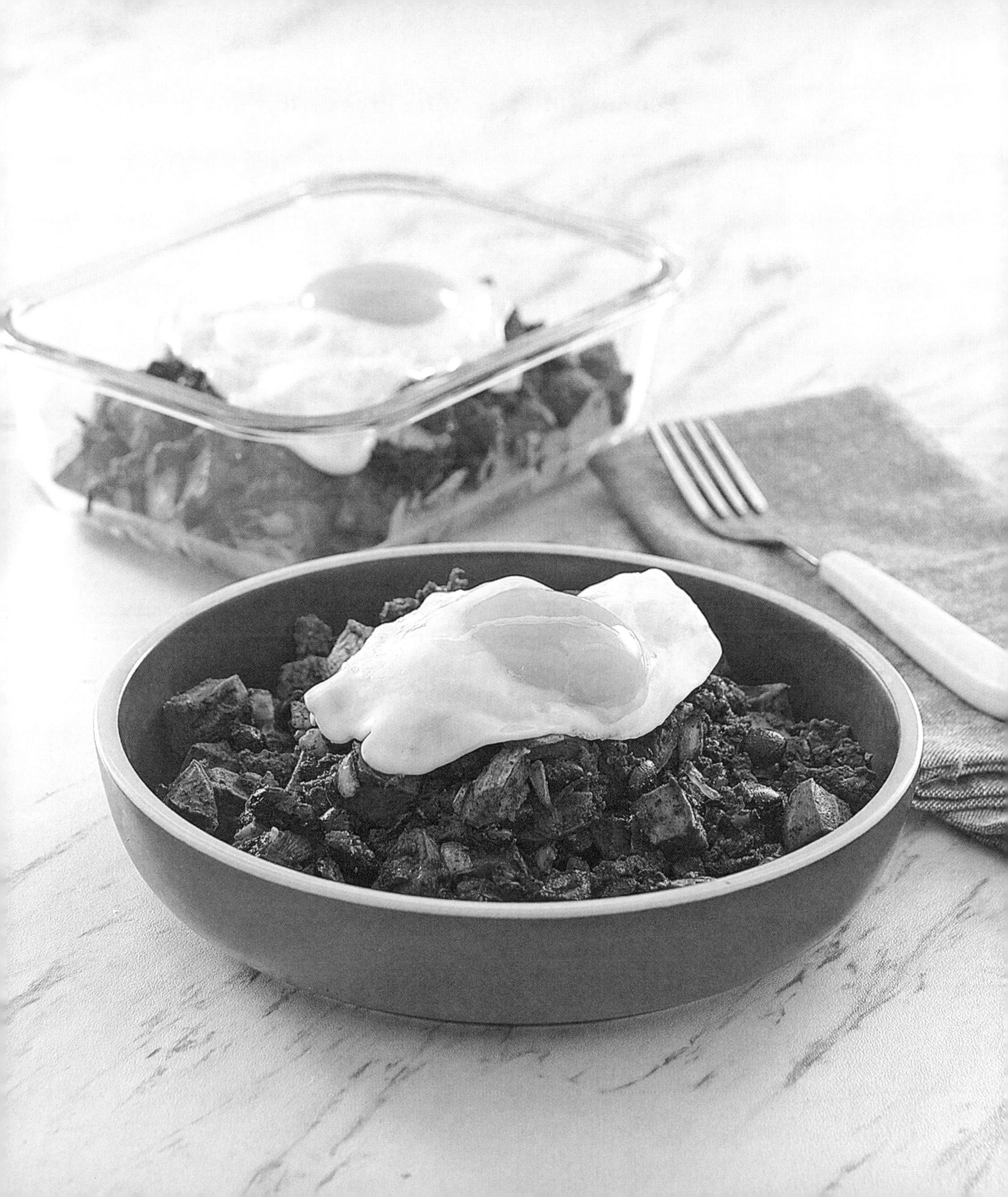

Peanut Butter Banana Protein Muffins

YIELDS 12 MUFFINS

Per Serving (1 muffin):

Calories	232
Fat	15g
Sodium	187mg
Carbohydrates	15g
Fiber	2g
Sugar	10g
Protein	11g

Thanks to the addition of protein powder, these muffins are as satiating as they are delicious. They make an excellent on-the-go breakfast, or you can keep them on hand for a quick snack in between meals.

2 large extra-ripe bananas

1 cup no-sugar-added creamy peanut butter

2 large eggs

¼ cup amber honey

¼ cup Tera's Whey vanilla protein powder

2 teaspoons vanilla extract

1 teaspoon baking powder

½ teaspoon sea salt

½ cup crushed peanuts

1. Preheat oven to 400°F. Line a twelve-cup muffin tin with paper or silicone cups.
2. Combine all ingredients, except peanuts, in a blender and blend until smooth. Stir in peanuts.
3. Pour equal amounts of batter into each muffin cup.
4. Bake 12 minutes or until a toothpick inserted in center comes out clean. Remove from oven and allow to cool 1 hour.
5. Store in an airtight container at room temperature up to 1 week.

Breakfast Burrito Bowls

One great thing about these burrito bowls is that they're fully customizable. You can use whatever vegetables you like or experiment with different seasoning mixtures to switch up the taste while still creating an easy meal. If you want to drop the fat, you can use lower-fat yogurt.

SERVES 6

Per Serving:

Calories	247
Fat	9g
Sodium	161mg
Carbohydrates	24g
Fiber	7g
Sugar	8g
Protein	17g

2 teaspoons avocado oil

8 ounces sweet potatoes, peeled and diced

1 large red bell pepper, seeded and diced

½ large yellow onion, peeled and finely chopped

1 (1.3-ounce) packet Siete Taco Seasoning

2 cups chopped kale

8 ounces white button mushrooms, finely chopped

1 teaspoon minced garlic

1 (15-ounce) can black beans, drained and rinsed

¾ cup full-fat plain Greek yogurt

6 large eggs, fried

1. Heat oil in a deep skillet over medium-high heat. Add sweet potatoes and cook 10 minutes or until they start to soften.
2. Add bell pepper, onion, and taco seasoning, stir, and continue to cook 15 minutes or until sweet potatoes are fork-tender.
3. Stir in kale, mushrooms, garlic, and beans and cook another 5 minutes. Remove from heat and allow to cool 20 minutes.
4. Divide equal parts vegetable mixture into six airtight containers. Top each with 2 tablespoons yogurt and a fried egg, cover, and store in refrigerator until ready to eat, up to 1 week.
5. Serve cold or heat in a skillet over medium-low heat 5 minutes or until warmed through.

Loaded Egg Bites

SERVES 6

Per Serving (4 egg bites):

Calories	224
Fat	16g
Sodium	404mg
Carbohydrates	4g
Fiber	1g
Sugar	1g
Protein	16g

Another versatile recipe, this high-protein breakfast allows you to take eggs with you on the go—and it takes only minutes to prep.

1 teaspoon avocado oil

1 medium green bell pepper, seeded and diced

½ large yellow onion, peeled and finely diced

1 teaspoon minced garlic

8 ounces ground pork

½ teaspoon sea salt

¼ teaspoon ground black pepper

¼ teaspoon ground sage

8 large eggs, lightly beaten

6 tablespoons crumbled feta cheese

1. Preheat oven to 350°F. Spray a twenty-four-cup mini muffin tin with avocado oil cooking spray.
2. Heat oil in a large skillet over medium heat. Add bell pepper and onion and cook 5 minutes or until vegetables start to soften.
3. Add garlic, pork, salt, pepper, and sage and cook until pork is no longer pink, about 7 minutes.
4. Transfer to a large mixing bowl and allow to cool 5 minutes. Add eggs and toss to combine.
5. Pour equal amounts of mixture into each muffin cup. Sprinkle ¾ teaspoon of feta on top of each.
6. Bake 10 minutes or until eggs are cooked through. Remove from oven and allow to cool 30 minutes before removing bites from muffin tin.
7. Store in an airtight container in refrigerator until ready to eat, up to 1 week. Reheat for 20 seconds in microwave before eating.

A TRICK FOR GETTING THE FLUFFIEST EGGS

Many people think the trick to getting fluffy eggs is to add a little milk before beating them, but there's actually a better way. Adding 1 tablespoon of plain seltzer water per egg will give you the airiest, fluffiest eggs you can imagine. That's because the bubbles in the seltzer create little pockets of air when heated, which makes the eggs lighter.

Spicy Sweet Potato and Sausage Hash

If you don't like your eggs runny, you can make this hash with hard-boiled eggs instead.

SERVES 6

Per Serving:

Calories	291
Fat	12g
Sodium	960mg
Carbohydrates	20g
Fiber	4g
Sugar	8g
Protein	24g

1 tablespoon avocado oil

2 medium sweet potatoes, peeled and diced

1 large yellow onion, peeled and finely chopped

1 large red bell pepper, seeded and diced

2 teaspoons garlic powder

1 teaspoon sea salt

½ teaspoon ground black pepper

½ teaspoon paprika

¼ teaspoon cayenne pepper

6 Applegate Organics Fire Roasted Red Pepper Chicken Sausage, diced

12 soft-boiled eggs, peeled

1. Heat oil in a large skillet over medium heat. Add sweet potatoes and cook 5 minutes. Add onion, bell pepper, garlic powder, salt, black pepper, paprika, and cayenne pepper and cook 2 more minutes. Add sausage and cook another 5 minutes or until sweet potatoes are tender. Remove from heat and allow to cool slightly, about 5 minutes.
2. Divide mixture evenly into each of six airtight containers. Top each with 2 eggs.
3. Cover and store in refrigerator until ready to eat, up to 1 week. When ready to serve, remove eggs, reheat in microwave or on stove, and then slice the eggs in half before serving.

Spinach and Artichoke Egg Casserole

SERVES 6

Per Serving:

Calories	258
Fat	16g
Sodium	754mg
Carbohydrates	9g
Fiber	2g
Sugar	2g
Protein	19g

This high-protein breakfast mimics your favorite spinach and artichoke dip, but with all whole ingredients and plenty of vegetables.

- **1 tablespoon extra-virgin olive oil**
- **½ medium yellow onion, peeled and finely diced**
- **1 teaspoon minced garlic**
- **6 cups packed fresh spinach, roughly chopped**
- **1½ cups drained jarred artichoke hearts**
- **1 teaspoon dried basil**
- **¼ teaspoon dried oregano**
- **½ teaspoon sea salt**
- **¼ teaspoon ground black pepper**
- **¼ teaspoon red pepper flakes**
- **1½ cups shredded mozzarella cheese, divided**
- **¼ cup grated Parmesan cheese, divided**
- **8 large eggs**
- **3 tablespoons organic half-and-half**

1. Preheat oven to 350°F. Spray an 8" × 8" baking dish with avocado oil cooking spray and set aside.
2. Heat oil in a large skillet over medium heat. Add onion and cook 2 minutes. Add garlic and cook an additional 3 minutes.
3. Stir in spinach and cook 3 minutes or until slightly wilted. Add artichoke hearts, basil, oregano, salt, black pepper, and red pepper flakes and cook another 2 minutes or until artichoke hearts are heated through. Remove from heat and spread out evenly in prepared baking dish. Layer ¾ cup mozzarella and 2 tablespoons Parmesan on top.
4. Add eggs and half-and-half to a large bowl and lightly whisk. Pour eggs on top of cheese. Sprinkle remaining ¾ cup mozzarella and remaining 2 tablespoons Parmesan on top.
5. Bake 30 minutes or until eggs are set and a knife inserted in center comes out clean. Remove from oven and allow to cool 1 hour.
6. Cut into six squares and transfer each square to an airtight container. Store in refrigerator until ready to eat, up to 1 week.
7. To serve, transfer to a skillet and cook over medium-low heat 5 minutes, or microwave 1 minute, or until heated through.

Basic Protein Waffles

These waffles are delicious as is, but you can also spread on some almond butter or other toppings, or use them as a high-protein bread for a breakfast sandwich.

SERVES 6

Per Serving (2 waffles):

Calories	126
Fat	2g
Sodium	212mg
Carbohydrates	18g
Fiber	2g
Sugar	4g
Protein	9g

1½ cups gluten-free rolled oats

1 cup cottage cheese

¾ cup egg whites

¾ cup frozen berries

1. Preheat waffle iron. Spray with avocado oil cooking spray.
2. Add oats, cottage cheese, and egg whites to a blender and blend until smooth.
3. Transfer to a large mixing bowl and stir in berries.
4. Scoop ¼ cup mixture onto waffle iron and cook 3 minutes or until waffle no longer sticks. Transfer to a large plate and repeat with remaining batter.
5. Allow to cool 20 minutes and transfer to a large, airtight container. Store at room temperature until ready to eat, up to 1 week.
6. Toast waffles before serving.

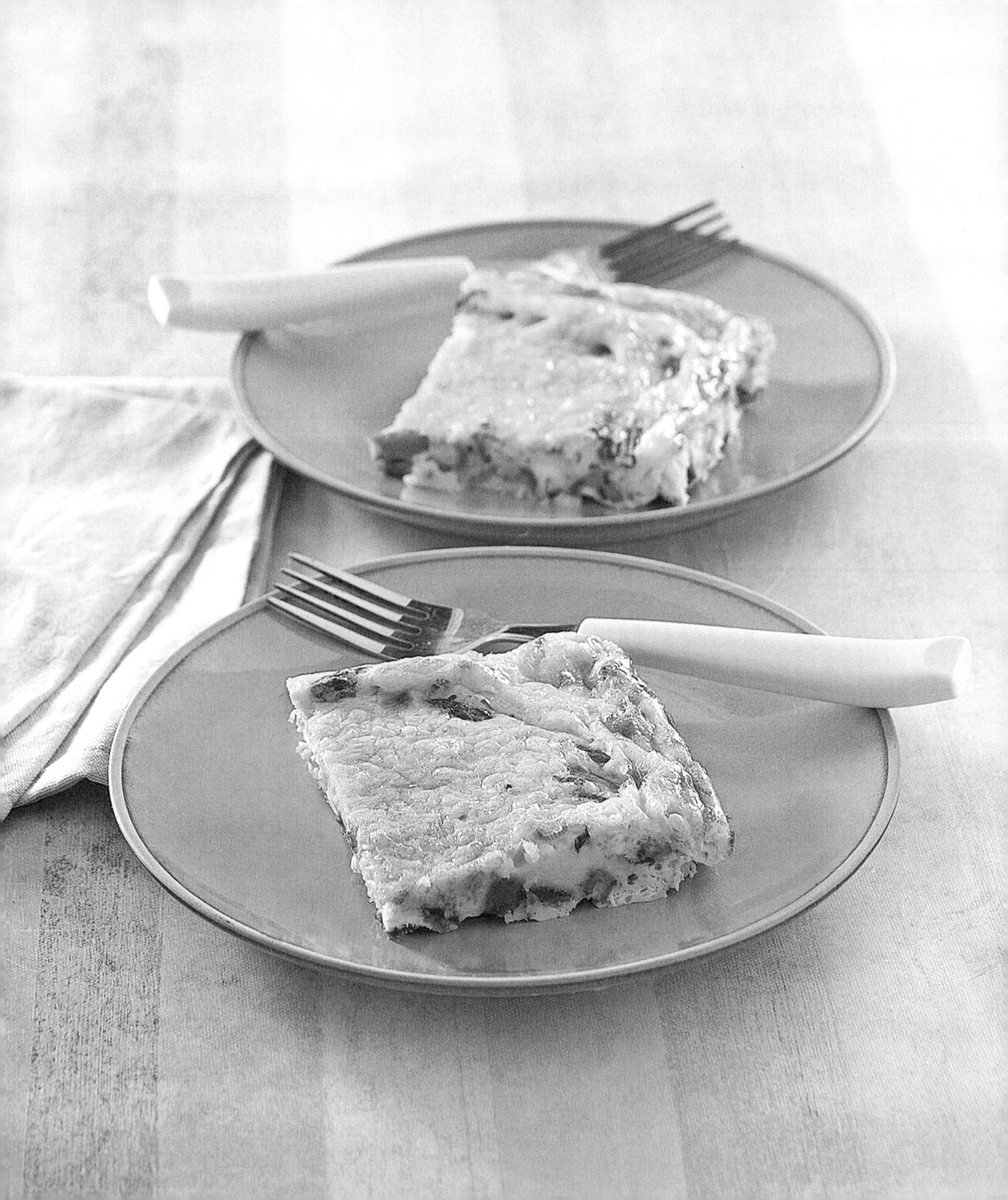

Bacon-Wrapped Asparagus Frittata

Bacon-wrapped asparagus is a summertime grilling favorite, but you can turn this flavor combo into a breakfast staple to have all year round. If the bacon adds too much fat for your macro allowance, feel free to cut back a little bit.

SERVES 6

Per Serving:

Calories	301
Fat	22g
Sodium	864mg
Carbohydrates	2g
Fiber	0g
Sugar	0g
Protein	24g

- 10 slices no-sugar-added bacon, roughly chopped
- 8 medium asparagus stalks, cut into ¼" pieces
- 1 teaspoon minced garlic
- 12 large eggs
- ¼ cup organic heavy cream
- 1 cup shredded Cheddar cheese, divided
- 2 tablespoons chopped scallions
- 1 teaspoon sea salt
- ½ teaspoon ground black pepper

1. Preheat oven to 350°F. Spray a 9" × 9" baking dish with avocado oil cooking spray.
2. Heat a large skillet over medium heat and add bacon. Cook 8 minutes or until crispy. Transfer bacon to a large paper towel–lined plate, reserving bacon grease in pan.
3. Add asparagus to pan with grease and cook 3 minutes or until it starts to soften. Add garlic and cook 1 more minute.
4. Add eggs and cream to a large mixing bowl and whisk lightly. Fold in cooked bacon and asparagus, ¾ cup cheese, scallions, salt, and pepper.
5. Transfer mixture to prepared baking dish. Sprinkle with remaining ¼ cup cheese and bake 20 minutes or until egg is set. Remove from oven and allow to cool 1 hour.
6. Cut into six pieces and transfer each piece to an airtight container. Store in refrigerator until ready to eat, up to 1 week.
7. Heat in microwave 20 seconds before serving.

REHEATING EGGS

The microwave is a quick way to reheat eggs, but if you have a little extra time, the best way to reheat a frittata is by baking it in the oven at 325°F for about 15 minutes or until heated through.

Freezer Breakfast Burritos

SERVES 6

Per Serving:

Calories	247
Fat	18g
Sodium	1,101mg
Carbohydrates	2g
Fiber	0g
Sugar	0g
Protein	22g

Frozen breakfast burritos are one of the most convenient breakfast options, but most packaged versions are filled with less-than-desirable ingredients. These homemade breakfast burritos, which are made with macro-friendly whole ingredients, keep in your freezer for up to three months so they're ready whenever you need them.

12 large eggs, lightly beaten

1 teaspoon sea salt

½ teaspoon ground black pepper

6 lavash flatbread wraps

12 slices no-sugar-added bacon, cooked

6 slices Cheddar cheese

¾ cup no-sugar-added salsa

1. Spray a large skillet with avocado oil cooking spray and heat over medium heat. Add eggs, salt, and pepper to hot pan and cook 7 minutes or until eggs are scrambled and fully cooked through. Remove from heat.
2. Lay each lavash flatbread on top of a piece of parchment paper. Add equal parts scrambled eggs to each flatbread. Layer 2 slices bacon, 1 slice cheese, and 2 tablespoons salsa on top of each portion.
3. Tightly roll up flatbread, forming a burrito. Wrap parchment paper around each burrito and secure with tape.
4. Place burritos in a freezer-safe bag and freeze until ready to eat, up to 3 months.
5. Before serving, remove burrito from parchment paper and microwave on high 90 seconds, or heat in oven at 350°F 10 minutes or until heated through.

Hash and Egg Bake

When making this egg bake, don't skip the step of letting the potatoes sweat first. If you do, you'll end up with a runny dish (that's still delicious, but not as portable).

SERVES 6

Per Serving:

Calories	177
Fat	10g
Sodium	923mg
Carbohydrates	11g
Fiber	1g
Sugar	1g
Protein	11g

2 medium white potatoes, peeled and shredded
1¼ teaspoons sea salt, divided
6 large eggs
¼ cup grated Parmesan cheese
½ cup unsweetened almond milk
1 teaspoon garlic powder
1 teaspoon onion powder
¼ teaspoon ground black pepper
1 cup chopped broccoli
½ cup shredded Cheddar cheese

1. Preheat oven to 350°F. Spray an 8" × 8" baking dish with avocado oil cooking spray.
2. Put potatoes in a strainer and sprinkle 1 teaspoon salt on top. Set aside to let sweat 10 minutes.
3. Add eggs, Parmesan, almond milk, garlic powder, onion powder, remaining ¼ teaspoon salt, and pepper to a large bowl and whisk until incorporated. Stir in broccoli.
4. Put potatoes in a cheesecloth or nut bag and squeeze out excess liquid. Spread potatoes out in prepared baking dish. Pour egg mixture on top. Sprinkle with Cheddar.
5. Bake 30 minutes or until eggs are set. Remove from oven and allow to cool 1 hour.
6. Cut into six pieces and store each piece in an airtight container in refrigerator until ready to eat, up to 1 week.
7. To serve, transfer to a baking dish and bake at 325°F 15 minutes, or microwave 1 minute, or until heated through.

HOW SWEATING WORKS

Adding salt to moisture-rich vegetables and letting them sit for a little while before cooking them is called "sweating." The salt has a hardening effect on the cellulose, part of the plant wall and a major fiber in vegetables, and helps pull out excess juices. Sweating also helps draw out flavor and soften the vegetables before fully cooking them.

Carrot Cake Breakfast "Cookies"

SERVES 6

Per Serving (2 cookies):

Calories	201
Fat	5g
Sodium	279mg
Carbohydrates	21g
Fiber	9g
Sugar	3g
Protein	19g

If you have some carbs to spare, you can add some raisins or Lily's stevia-sweetened chocolate chips to the batter right before baking these protein-rich cookies.

1 cup gluten-free rolled oats
2 scoops Tera's Whey vanilla protein powder
6 tablespoons coconut flour
1 teaspoon ground cinnamon
½ teaspoon ground nutmeg
¼ teaspoon sea salt
1 tablespoon Nutiva Buttery Flavor Coconut Oil, melted
2 large egg whites
2 teaspoons vanilla extract
2 tablespoons ChocZero Maple-Flavored Syrup
1 cup peeled shredded carrots

1. Preheat oven to 325°F. Line a baking sheet with parchment paper.
2. Combine oats, protein powder, coconut flour, cinnamon, nutmeg, and salt in a large bowl.
3. Add coconut oil, egg whites, vanilla, and maple syrup and fold until just combined. Fold in shredded carrots.
4. Use a small cookie scoop to scoop 2 tablespoons dough onto prepared baking sheet. Repeat with remaining batter, spacing out scoops on sheet.
5. Bake 10 minutes or until cookies are set. Remove from oven and allow to cool 1 hour on sheet.
6. Transfer to an airtight container and store in refrigerator until ready to eat, up to 1 week. Allow to come to room temperature before enjoying.

Macro-Friendly Banana Bread

This high-protein banana bread is an easy-to-eat and filling option when you must take breakfast on the go, or you just want to eat something without a lot of fuss. If you want to drop the carbs a bit, you can swap the maple syrup for a stevia-sweetened version. You can also opt for gluten-free pancake mix, but keep in mind that might drop the protein significantly.

SERVES 6

Per Serving (1 slice):

Calories	257
Fat	10g
Sodium	183mg
Carbohydrates	34g
Fiber	7g
Sugar	13g
Protein	9g

2 large eggs

3 large ripe bananas, mashed

2 tablespoons Nutiva Buttery Flavor Coconut Oil, melted

2 tablespoons pure maple syrup

1 teaspoon vanilla extract

1¼ cups Kodiak Cakes Protein-Packed Flapjack and Waffle Mix

1½ teaspoons baking powder

1 teaspoon ground cinnamon

¼ teaspoon ground nutmeg

½ cup Lily's stevia-sweetened chocolate chips

1. Preheat oven to 350°F. Line an 8" × 4" loaf pan with parchment paper.
2. Add eggs, bananas, coconut oil, maple syrup, and vanilla to a large bowl and whisk until smooth.
3. Add pancake mix, baking powder, cinnamon, and nutmeg and stir until just combined. Fold in chocolate chips.
4. Transfer batter to prepared pan and bake 30 minutes or until toothpick inserted in center comes out clean. Remove from oven and allow to cool 1 hour.
5. Cut into six large slices or twelve thinner slices. Transfer to an airtight container and store at room temperature until ready to eat, up to 1 week.

Sheet Pan Frittata

SERVES 6

Per Serving:

Calories	300
Fat	19g
Sodium	798mg
Carbohydrates	12g
Fiber	3g
Sugar	5g
Protein	22g

This frittata is not only versatile ingredient-wise; there are a lot of serving possibilities too. You can eat it as is, roll up a piece in a tortilla or serve it on top of roasted sweet potatoes if you have some carbs to spare, or throw it on top of a salad for some extra protein.

1 medium head broccoli, chopped into florets

1 pint cherry tomatoes, halved

1 teaspoon extra-virgin olive oil

1½ teaspoons sea salt, divided

12 large eggs

1 cup 2% organic milk

½ teaspoon ground black pepper

1 cup shredded Cheddar cheese

1. Preheat oven to 375°F. Line a rimmed baking sheet with parchment paper.
2. Spread out broccoli and tomatoes on prepared baking sheet, drizzle oil on top, and sprinkle with ½ teaspoon salt.
3. Roast 20 minutes or until broccoli is tender and slightly charred.
4. While vegetables are cooking, add eggs, milk, remaining 1 teaspoon salt, and pepper to a large bowl and whisk.
5. Pour eggs on top of cooked vegetables. Sprinkle cheese over eggs.
6. Bake 30 minutes or until eggs are set. Remove from oven and allow to cool 30 minutes.
7. Cut into twelve squares and transfer two squares into each of six airtight containers. Store in refrigerator until ready to eat, up to 1 week.
8. To serve, transfer to a baking dish and bake at 325°F 15 minutes or in microwave 1 minute or until heated through.

Cottage Cheese Muffins

Cottage cheese is a protein-packed ingredient, but some people don't care for the flavor. Even if you fall into that camp, you'll love these muffins. You'll get all of the filling benefits without even tasting the cottage cheese.

SERVES 6

Per Serving (2 muffins):

Calories	360
Fat	24g
Sodium	336mg
Carbohydrates	12g
Fiber	4g
Sugar	4g
Protein	24g

1¼ cups full-fat cottage cheese
5 large eggs
¼ cup 2% organic milk
1½ cups almond flour
⅓ cup chickpea flour
1 teaspoon baking powder
½ cup shredded mozzarella cheese
1 cup chopped cooked broccoli florets
¼ cup grated Cheddar cheese
⅓ cup chopped scallions

1. Preheat oven to 400°F. Line a twelve-cup muffin tin with paper or silicone cups.
2. Add cottage cheese, eggs, and milk to a large bowl and whisk until combined. Stir in almond flour, chickpea flour, and baking powder.
3. Add mozzarella and broccoli and toss to combine.
4. Scoop even amounts of mixture into each muffin cup. Sprinkle Cheddar and scallions on top.
5. Bake 30 minutes or until set. Remove from oven and allow to cool 30 minutes.
6. Remove muffins from tin and transfer two to each of six airtight containers. Store in refrigerator until ready to eat, up to 1 week.
7. Allow to come to room temperature before serving.

PROTEIN IN COTTAGE CHEESE

Cottage cheese is a powerhouse ingredient for the macro diet because it has a whopping 25 grams of protein per cup. Like other dairy products, it's also available in different fat percentages so you can pick the one that works best for your meal plan.

CHAPTER 3

Salads and Bowls

Quinoa and Black Bean Power Bowls

SERVES 6

Per Serving:

Calories	421
Fat	17g
Sodium	402mg
Carbohydrates	53g
Fiber	12g
Sugar	2g
Protein	14g

WHY CHOOSE SPROUTED GRAINS?

One downside to grains is that they contain anti-nutrients, or compounds that prevent you from properly absorbing vitamins and minerals. They can also be hard to digest. Sprouting, also called germinating, involves soaking grains in water for one to five days. This breaks down some of the starch and phytates (anti-nutrients), making the nutrients more bioavailable and making the grains easier to digest. You can sprout any grains yourself, but many manufacturers (such as Thrive Market and TruRoots) sell them already sprouted.

These vegetarian power bowls have plenty of protein as is, but if you want to up the grams significantly, you can add chicken, ground beef, ground turkey, or your favorite high-quality meat.

2 medium sweet potatoes, peeled and cut into 1" cubes
2 tablespoons avocado oil
½ teaspoon sea salt
½ teaspoon ground cumin
2 tablespoons hemp seeds
1 (15-ounce) can black beans, drained and rinsed
1½ cups cooked sprouted quinoa
3 cups chopped kale
6 tablespoons tahini

1. Preheat oven to 400°F. Line a baking sheet with parchment paper.
2. Add sweet potato cubes to a large bowl, drizzle with oil, and season with salt and cumin. Toss to evenly coat. Spread sweet potatoes out evenly on prepared baking sheet.
3. Roast 20 minutes, then remove from oven and add hemp seeds and beans. Spread out evenly and return to oven for 10 minutes. Remove from oven and allow to cool 20 minutes.
4. Scoop ¼ cup quinoa into each of six airtight containers. Top each with ½ cup kale and equal parts sweet potato and bean mixture.
5. Drizzle each portion with 1 tablespoon tahini or store tahini in a separate container and add it right before eating. Store in refrigerator until ready to eat, up to 1 week. Serve cold.

Spicy Tuna Bowls

These macro-friendly bowls can be easily customized based on your specific goals. If you want to lower the carbs, you can skip the brown rice and add lettuce right before eating.

SERVES 6

Per Serving:

Calories	239
Fat	9g
Sodium	414mg
Carbohydrates	21g
Fiber	2g
Sugar	1g
Protein	18g

2 (5-ounce) cans solid white albacore tuna packed in water, drained

2 tablespoons Tessemae's Mayonnaise

1 tablespoon Dijon mustard

2 tablespoons sriracha

2 tablespoons chopped red onion

3 cups cooked brown rice

1 medium cucumber, diced

1 medium avocado, pitted, peeled, and sliced

6 tablespoons crumbled feta cheese

1. Add tuna, mayonnaise, mustard, sriracha, and onion to a large bowl. Mash until combined.
2. Scoop ½ cup brown rice into each of six airtight containers. Top each with equal parts tuna mixture, cucumber, and avocado and 1 tablespoon feta. Cover and store in refrigerator until ready to eat, up to 6 days. Serve cold.

Plant-Based Power Bowls

SERVES 6

Per Serving:

Calories	307
Fat	10g
Sodium	941mg
Carbohydrates	43g
Fiber	11g
Sugar	8g
Protein	13g

MAKE YOUR OWN VEGETABLE BROTH

Boxed vegetable broth is convenient, but many brands have added sugar. To make your own, sauté 1 medium onion (diced), 4 cloves garlic (minced), 4 large carrots (diced), and 4 medium stalks celery (diced) over medium-high heat 5 minutes. Add 10 cups water, 1 teaspoon salt, 2 teaspoons dried thyme, 2 teaspoons dried rosemary, 5 tablespoons tomato paste, 1 cup chopped kale, and 2 bay leaves. Bring to a boil, then reduce heat to low and simmer 1 hour. Strain and discard solids. Use right away or portion into 1-cup containers and freeze up to 6 months.

These hearty bowls are vegan-friendly, but if you eat meat and want to up the protein, you can add your favorite protein source. This is a time when having a bunch of shredded chicken already cooked will come in handy.

2 (15-ounce) cans chickpeas, drained and rinsed
1 teaspoon avocado oil
1 teaspoon paprika
2 teaspoons ground turmeric, divided
½ cup sprouted quinoa
1 cup vegetable broth
6 cups chopped kale
2 teaspoons extra-virgin olive oil
1 teaspoon sea salt
½ teaspoon ground black pepper
¾ cup shredded radishes
1 large avocado, peeled, pitted, and sliced
2 teaspoons fresh lemon juice

1. Preheat oven to 400°F.
2. Put chickpeas in a large bowl and drizzle with avocado oil. Sprinkle paprika and 1 teaspoon turmeric on top. Toss to coat evenly.
3. Spread out chickpeas on an ungreased baking sheet and roast 25 minutes. Remove from oven.
4. While chickpeas are roasting, combine quinoa, remaining 1 teaspoon turmeric, and broth in a medium saucepan. Bring to a boil over medium-high heat, then reduce heat to low. Cover and cook 15 minutes. Remove from heat and let sit, covered, 5 more minutes. Fluff with a fork.
5. Combine kale and olive oil in a large bowl and massage with your hands until kale starts to soften. Sprinkle with salt and pepper. Transfer 1 cup kale to each of six airtight containers.
6. Top kale with ¼ cup quinoa, equal parts chickpeas, 2 tablespoons radishes, and equal parts avocado. Drizzle lemon juice on top (mostly on avocado). Cover and store in refrigerator until ready to eat, up to 1 week. Serve cold.

Deconstructed Gyro Bowls

This recipe is a great way to repurpose any leftover Instant Pot® Beef Gyros from Chapter 6. You can make a big batch, eat some with warm pita or wrapped in lavash, and then make these bowls with the rest for fewer carbs in your week.

SERVES 6

Per Serving:

Calories	321
Fat	23g
Sodium	1,057mg
Carbohydrates	13g
Fiber	2g
Sugar	7g
Protein	21g

3 cups cooked cauliflower rice

1 batch Instant Pot® Beef Gyros with Tzatziki Sauce (see recipe in Chapter 6)

1½ cups halved cherry tomatoes

6 tablespoons minced red onion

1½ cups diced cucumbers

¾ cup chopped kalamata olives

¾ cup crumbled feta cheese

1. Scoop ½ cup cauliflower rice into each of six airtight containers. Top with equal parts Instant Pot® Beef Gyros with Tzatziki Sauce.
2. Add ¼ cup tomatoes, 1 tablespoon onion, ¼ cup cucumbers, 2 tablespoons olives, and 2 tablespoons feta to each container. Cover and store in refrigerator until ready to eat, up to 1 week. Serve cold.

Happy Gut Buddha Bowls

SERVES 6

Per Serving:

Calories	372
Fat	9g
Sodium	1,045mg
Carbohydrates	39g
Fiber	3g
Sugar	5g
Protein	33g

If you want to make this recipe vegetarian, you can opt for a plant protein source, like beans, chickpeas, or tofu instead. The total protein may drop a little bit, but you can make up for it with another meal or protein-rich snack.

FOR BOWLS

3 cups cooked sprouted brown rice

2 tablespoons extra-virgin olive oil

1 tablespoon apple cider vinegar

3 cups chopped kale

1½ pounds boneless, skinless chicken breasts, cooked and cut into bite-sized pieces

3 cups Wildbrine Korean Kimchi

1½ cups sliced radishes

6 tablespoons Cedar's Harissa Hummus

FOR SAUCE

3 tablespoons coconut aminos

2 tablespoons miso paste

3 cloves garlic, peeled and finely minced

½ teaspoon ground black pepper

⅛ teaspoon red pepper flakes

1. To make Bowls: Scoop ½ cup rice into each of six airtight containers.
2. Combine oil and vinegar in a small bowl. Pour over kale in a large bowl and massage 1 minute or until kale starts to soften. Push rice aside and add ½ cup kale to each container.
3. Top kale with equal parts chicken, ½ cup kimchi, ¼ cup radishes, and 1 tablespoon hummus.
4. To make Sauce: Whisk all ingredients in a small bowl. Pour 1 tablespoon Sauce into each of six small containers. Place small containers in Bowl containers, cover, and store in refrigerator until ready to eat, up to 1 week.
5. When ready to serve, pour Sauce over Bowl.

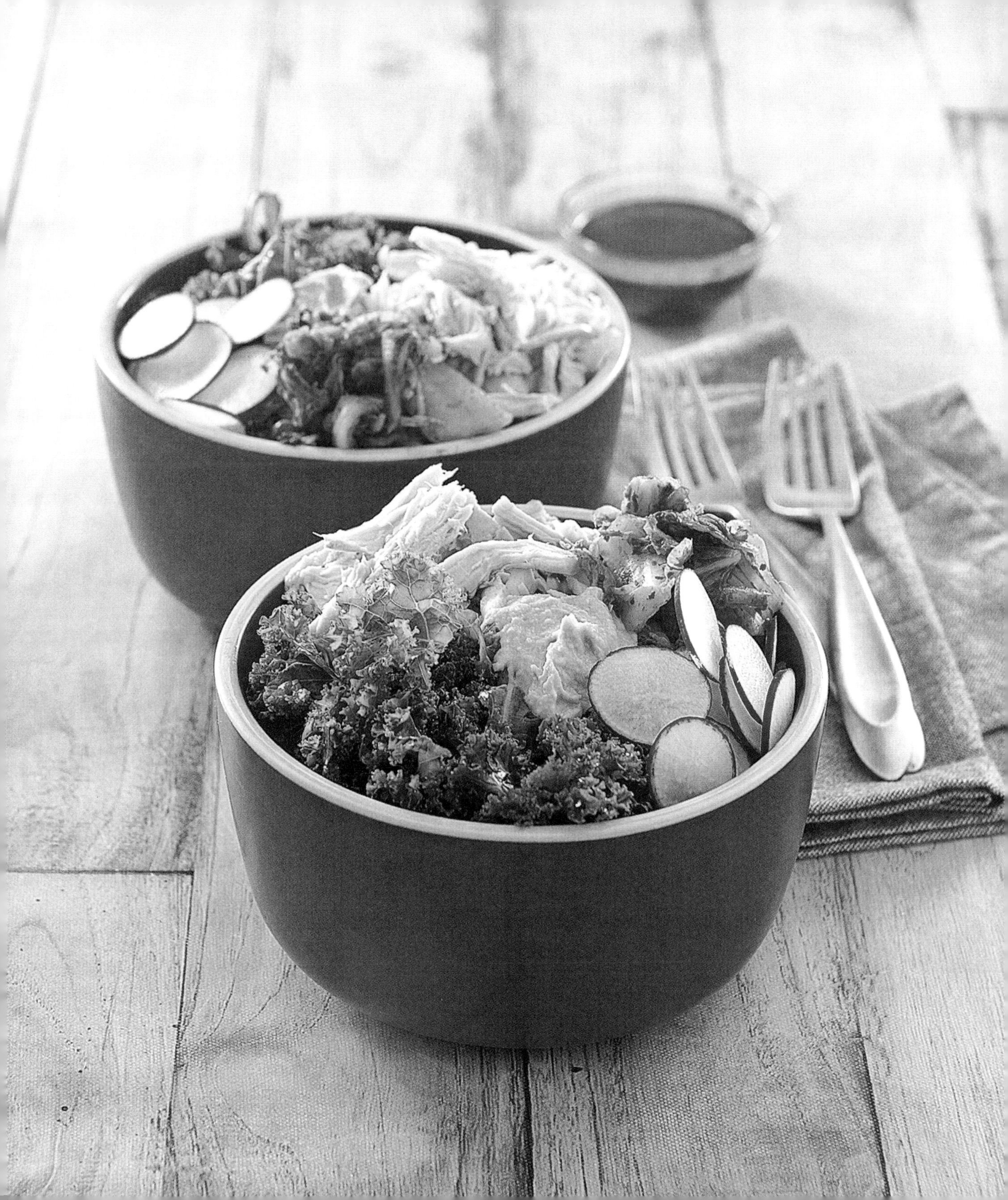

Miso Chicken Bowl

SERVES 6

Per Serving:

Calories	311
Fat	11g
Sodium	614mg
Carbohydrates	33g
Fiber	11g
Sugar	4g
Protein	20g

WHAT IS MISO?

Miso is a fermented paste that's made by combining soy with mold. As unappetizing as that sounds, miso is the ultimate umami flavor for dishes. It imparts a robust savory taste that has small hints of sweetness. Plus, since it's fermented, it's full of probiotics that support your gut health. Specifically, it contains *Aspergillus oryzae*, which can reduce the risk of inflammatory bowel disease and other digestive diseases.

If you need to drop the fat in this recipe, you can replace the chicken thighs with boneless, skinless chicken breasts. You can also use a lean steak, like strips of sirloin, instead of chicken to switch things up.

FOR CHICKEN

3 tablespoons ChocZero Maple-Flavored Syrup

1 tablespoon toasted sesame oil

1 tablespoon coconut aminos

1 tablespoon white miso paste

2 cloves garlic, peeled and minced

1½ pounds boneless, skinless chicken thighs, cut into bite-sized pieces

2 teaspoons avocado oil

FOR BOWLS

1½ cups sliced shiitake mushrooms

3 cups cooked brown rice

3 cups steamed broccoli florets

6 tablespoons toasted sesame seeds

¾ cup Noble Made Carrot Ginger Dressing

1. To make Chicken: In a large bowl, whisk together maple syrup, sesame oil, coconut aminos, miso paste, and garlic. Add chicken and toss to coat.
2. Heat avocado oil in a large skillet over medium-high heat. Add chicken and cook 7 minutes or until chicken is cooked through, browning on all sides. Scoop chicken out of pan with a slotted spoon and transfer equal parts to each of six airtight containers.
3. To make Bowls: Add mushrooms to hot skillet and cook 5 minutes or until mushrooms are softened but not mushy. Transfer ¼ cup cooked mushrooms to each container.
4. Top each container with ½ cup rice, ½ cup broccoli, 1 tablespoon sesame seeds, and 2 tablespoons dressing. Cover and store in refrigerator until ready to eat, up to 1 week. Serve cold.

Chicken and Quinoa Power Bowls

These power bowls are easy to customize—just switch out the protein and starches. You can use cooked ground beef or turkey, steak, or your favorite fish in place of the chicken, and swap out the quinoa for rice, or cauliflower rice if you want to lower the carbs. If you need to add some carbs, just throw in some roasted sweet potatoes.

SERVES 6

Per Serving:

Calories	423
Fat	14g
Sodium	334mg
Carbohydrates	33g
Fiber	8g
Sugar	5g
Protein	42g

FOR BOWLS

3 cups cooked sprouted quinoa

3 cups shredded cooked boneless, skinless chicken breasts

3 cups snap peas

1½ cups peeled shredded carrots

1½ cups finely chopped cabbage

6 tablespoons minced red onion

FOR SAUCE

½ cup tahini

2 tablespoons lemon juice

1 tablespoon chopped fresh parsley

2 cloves garlic, peeled and minced

½ teaspoon sea salt

1. To make Bowls: Scoop ½ cup quinoa, ½ cup chicken, ½ cup peas, ¼ cup carrots, ¼ cup cabbage, and 1 tablespoon onion each into six airtight containers.
2. To make Sauce: Whisk all ingredients in a medium bowl until smooth. Scoop 2 tablespoons Sauce into each of six small containers. Place small containers in Bowl containers, cover, and store in refrigerator until ready to eat, up to 1 week.
3. When ready to serve, pour Sauce over Bowl.

THE SCOOP ON TAHINI

Tahini, which is made from ground toasted sesame seeds, is a staple in Mediterranean and Middle Eastern cuisines. It's one of the main ingredients in hummus, and can be used in place of peanut butter or other nut butter in almost any recipe. Tahini also makes a great base for sauce to drizzle on power bowls and Buddha bowls.

Turkey Burrito Bowls

SERVES 6

Per Serving:

Calories	341
Fat	20g
Sodium	921mg
Carbohydrates	14g
Fiber	2g
Sugar	4g
Protein	27g

If you don't have Siete Taco Seasoning, you can use any macro-friendly taco seasoning of your choice. Check the ingredients and try to stay away from added sugar, a common hidden ingredient in lots of packaged seasonings.

2 teaspoons avocado oil, divided

1½ pounds 90% lean ground turkey

1 (1.3-ounce) packet Siete Taco Seasoning

1 small yellow onion, peeled and minced

4 cloves garlic, peeled and minced

1 (10-ounce) bag frozen cauliflower rice

1 (4.5-ounce) can fire-roasted green chiles, including juice

2 tablespoons tomato paste

1 teaspoon sea salt

1 teaspoon ground cumin

½ teaspoon ground black pepper

¼ teaspoon paprika

⅛ teaspoon cayenne pepper

6 tablespoons sour cream

¾ cup shredded sharp Cheddar cheese

6 tablespoons chopped black olives

6 tablespoons crushed plantain chips

1. Heat 1 teaspoon oil in a large skillet over medium-high heat. Crumble turkey into pan and cook 4 minutes. Sprinkle taco seasoning over meat and continue cooking until no longer pink, about 4 more minutes. Set aside.
2. Heat remaining 1 teaspoon oil in a separate large skillet over medium-high heat. Add onion and cook 5 minutes. Add garlic and cook another 1 minute.
3. Stir in cauliflower, green chiles with juice, tomato paste, salt, cumin, black pepper, paprika, and cayenne pepper. Cook 8 minutes or until cauliflower is softened.
4. Divide cauliflower into six equal portions. Scoop each portion into a separate airtight container. Top with equal parts turkey, 1 tablespoon sour cream, 2 tablespoons cheese, 1 tablespoon olives, and 1 tablespoon plantain chips. Cover and store in refrigerator until ready to eat, up to 1 week. Serve cold.

Fall Harvest Bowls

If you don't want to add raw beets to these bowls, you can substitute a beet sauerkraut like the Wildbrine Red Beet & Cabbage Organic Kraut. Technically, it's still raw, but the fermentation process makes it a little softer, and it adds loads of probiotics to help your gut health.

SERVES 6

Per Serving:

Calories	405
Fat	20g
Sodium	438mg
Carbohydrates	20g
Fiber	5g
Sugar	4g
Protein	36g

FOR BOWLS

- 3 cups peeled cubed sweet potato
- 3 cups peeled cubed pumpkin
- 2 teaspoons extra-virgin olive oil
- ½ teaspoon sea salt
- ½ teaspoon ground black pepper
- ¼ teaspoon paprika
- 3 cups shredded cooked boneless, skinless chicken breasts
- 1½ cups cooked sprouted brown rice
- 1½ cups canned chickpeas, drained and rinsed
- 1½ cups shredded beets
- 1½ cups pumpkin seeds

FOR SAUCE

- ¼ cup tahini
- 2 tablespoons extra-virgin olive oil
- 2 tablespoons lemon juice
- 1 tablespoon water
- 1 tablespoon ChocZero Maple-Flavored Syrup
- 1 clove garlic, peeled and minced
- ½ teaspoon sea salt

1. Preheat oven to 400°F. Line a baking sheet with parchment paper.
2. To make Bowls: Spread out sweet potato and pumpkin in a single layer on prepared baking sheet. Drizzle with oil, then sprinkle with salt, pepper, and paprika. Roast 40 minutes or until tender and starting to turn golden brown. Remove from oven and allow to cool 20 minutes.
3. Scoop ½ cup sweet potato, ½ cup pumpkin, ½ cup chicken, ¼ cup rice, ¼ cup chickpeas, ¼ cup beets, and ¼ cup pumpkin seeds into each of six airtight containers.
4. To make Sauce: Whisk together all ingredients in a small bowl. Pour 2 tablespoons into each of six small containers. Place Sauce containers in Bowl containers, cover, and store in refrigerator until ready to eat, up to 1 week.
5. When ready to serve, pour Sauce over Bowl.

Green Goddess Bowls

SERVES 6

Per Serving:

Calories	460
Fat	21g
Sodium	441mg
Carbohydrates	30g
Fiber	6g
Sugar	4g
Protein	37g

A+ FOR ARUGULA

Arugula is a bitter green that has a sort of peppery taste. Like broccoli, it's classified as a cruciferous vegetable, which means it's loaded with micronutrients, like vitamins A, C, and K, plus magnesium and folate. One benefit of leafy greens is that you get a lot of micronutrients without a significant amount of macronutrients or calories, so you can work them into most meals without throwing off the macros.

If you want to make sure the arugula stays fresh and crispy when you eat your Green Goddess Bowl, keep it in a separate container and add it right before eating, rather than storing it with the other ingredients.

FOR BOWLS

- 3 cups snap peas, ends trimmed
- 24 medium asparagus spears, ends trimmed
- 3 cups cooked sprouted quinoa
- 3 (6-ounce) cans wild pink salmon, drained
- 1½ cups chopped cucumber
- 1½ cups pumpkin seeds
- 6 cups arugula

FOR DRESSING

- ½ cup 2% plain Greek yogurt
- 1 tablespoon lemon juice
- ½ teaspoon grated lemon zest
- 2 teaspoons extra-virgin olive oil
- 2 cloves garlic, peeled and minced
- ¼ cup chopped fresh dill
- ½ teaspoon sea salt
- ¼ teaspoon ground black pepper

1. To make Bowls: Bring a large pot of water to a boil over high heat. Add peas and asparagus and cook 3 minutes or until slightly softened. Drain water and set aside.
2. Scoop ½ cup quinoa into each of six airtight containers. Top with ½ cup peas, 4 asparagus spears, ½ can salmon, ¼ cup cucumber, and ¼ cup pumpkin seeds. Top with 1 cup arugula.
3. To make Dressing: Whisk all ingredients in a small bowl. Scoop 2 tablespoons Dressing into each of six small containers. Place small containers in Bowl containers, cover, and store in refrigerator until ready to eat, up to 1 week.
4. When ready to serve, pour Dressing over Bowl.

Spicy Cajun Bowls

These Spicy Cajun Bowls pack some serious heat. If you like the idea but need to dial it down a bit, you can reduce the Cajun seasoning by half and still get an excellent, albeit less spicy, result.

SERVES 6

Per Serving:

Calories	283
Fat	3g
Sodium	782mg
Carbohydrates	29g
Fiber	2g
Sugar	3g
Protein	33g

2 teaspoons extra-virgin olive oil, divided

1½ pounds boneless, skinless chicken breasts, cut into 1" cubes

2 teaspoons Slap Ya Mama Cajun Seasoning

1 large red bell pepper, seeded and diced

1 (15-ounce) can black beans, drained and rinsed

¾ teaspoon sea salt

½ teaspoon ground black pepper

½ teaspoon paprika

3 cups roasted peeled cubed sweet potatoes

1. Heat 1 teaspoon oil in a large skillet over medium-high heat. Add chicken and cook 2 minutes. Sprinkle with Cajun seasoning and continue to cook 6 minutes or until chicken is no longer pink.
2. Scoop chicken out of pan with a slotted spoon and divide equally into six airtight containers.
3. Heat remaining 1 teaspoon oil in skillet and add bell pepper. Cook 4 minutes or until pepper starts to soften. Stir in beans and cook 1 minute or until heated through. Sprinkle with salt, pepper, and paprika and cook 1 more minute.
4. Scoop equal parts bean mixture into each container with chicken. Add ½ cup sweet potatoes to each container. Cover and store in refrigerator until ready to eat, up to 1 week. Serve cold.

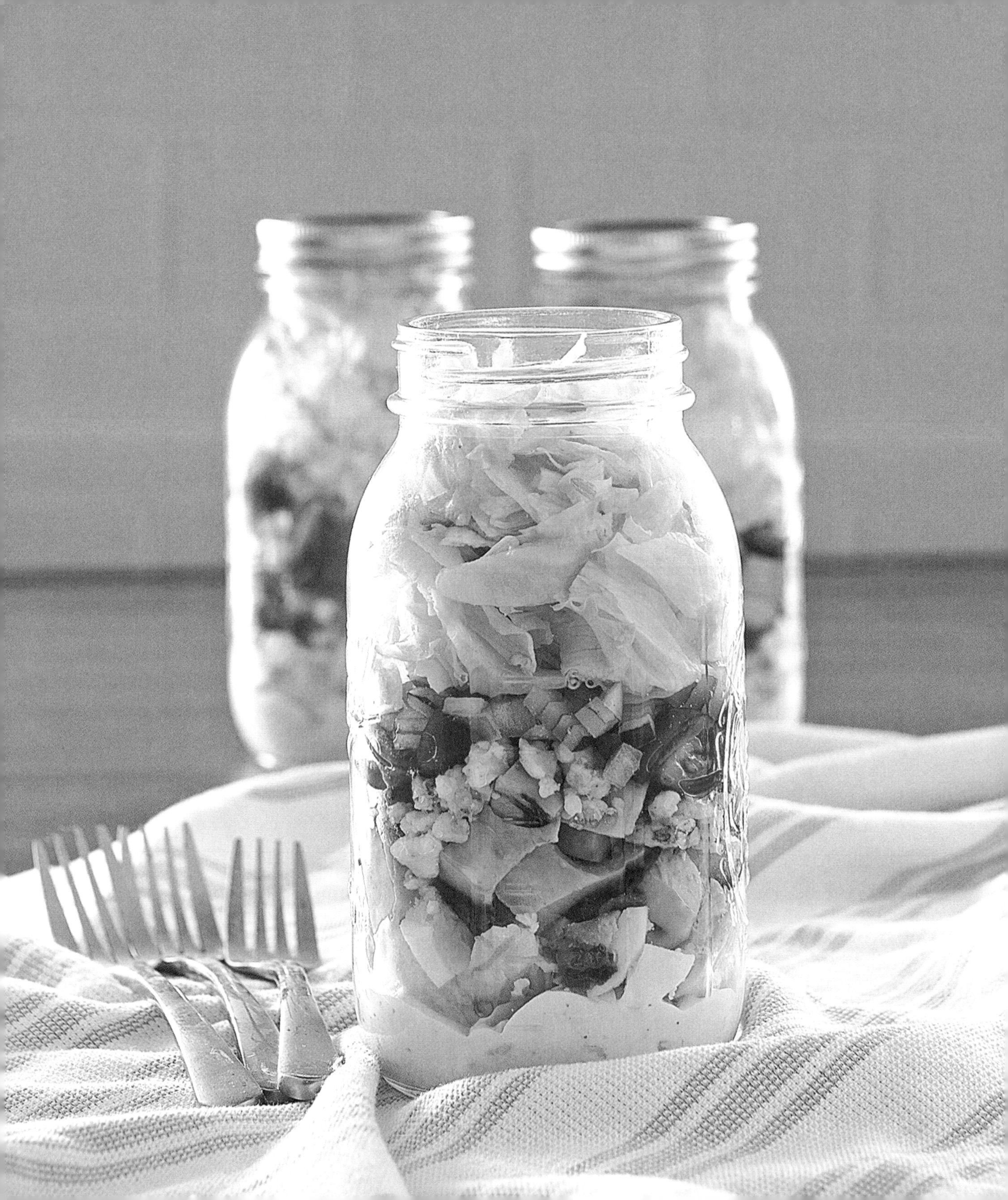

Mason Jar Cobb Salad

This Mason Jar Cobb Salad is loaded with protein and healthy fats. If you want to add some more carbs, you can throw in some roasted sweet potato or chickpeas, which also have a considerable amount of fiber.

SERVES 6

Per Serving:

Calories	597
Fat	43g
Sodium	1,123mg
Carbohydrates	6g
Fiber	2g
Sugar	2g
Protein	46g

¾ cup Tessemae's Creamy Ranch Dressing

3 cups shredded cooked boneless, skinless chicken breasts

¾ cup chopped hard-boiled eggs

¾ cup chopped cooked no-sugar-added bacon

¾ cup chopped avocado

¾ cup crumbled blue cheese

¾ cup chopped grape tomatoes

6 tablespoons minced red onion

6 cups chopped iceberg lettuce

1. Put 2 tablespoons dressing in the bottom of each of six quart-sized Mason jars.
2. Layer ½ cup chicken, 2 tablespoons eggs, 2 tablespoons bacon, 2 tablespoons avocado, 2 tablespoons blue cheese, 2 tablespoons tomato, 1 tablespoon onion, and 1 cup lettuce in each jar.
3. Store in refrigerator until ready to eat, up to 1 week. When ready to serve, shake vigorously.

BLT Salad with Chicken

SERVES 6

Per Serving:

Calories	508
Fat	35g
Sodium	730mg
Carbohydrates	6g
Fiber	4g
Sugar	2g
Protein	42g

This BLT salad is a bit higher in fat than most of the other salads, so make sure you're working it in on days when you're eating lower-fat meals. If you want to reduce the fat a bit, you can use just 1 tablespoon of dressing in each jar or scale back on the bacon. Try to keep the avocado though!

3⁄4 cup Tessemae's Mayonnaise
1½ teaspoons lemon juice
1 tablespoon minced scallions
¼ teaspoon sea salt
¼ teaspoon ground black pepper
3⁄4 cup chopped cooked no-sugar-added bacon
3 cups chopped cooked boneless, skinless chicken breasts
1½ cups chopped Roma tomatoes
1½ cups chopped avocado
6 cups chopped iceberg lettuce

1. Add mayonnaise, lemon juice, scallions, salt, and pepper to a small bowl and whisk until smooth. Scoop 2 tablespoons into each of six wide-mouth quart-sized Mason jars.
2. Layer 2 tablespoons bacon, ½ cup chicken, ¼ cup tomato, ¼ cup avocado, and 1 cup lettuce in each jar. Cover and refrigerate until ready to eat, up to 1 week.
3. When ready to serve, shake vigorously.

THE GOOD FAT IN AVOCADOS

Avocados are technically classified as a fruit, but they're one of the only fruits that contain a significant amount of fat. Because of this, they count heavily toward your fat macros, but they're worth it. They've been shown to help lower LDL (or "bad") cholesterol and reduce your risk of heart disease and/or stroke. If you want to keep your avocados from browning in your prepped meals, squeeze a little fresh lemon juice on them.

Barbecue Ranch Chicken Salad

When making your barbecue chicken, you might want to consider doubling or tripling the recipe. It freezes well and makes a great protein-rich meal combined with easy sides like brown rice, quinoa, cauliflower rice, or a salad.

SERVES 6

Per Serving:

Calories	302
Fat	21g
Sodium	246mg
Carbohydrates	13g
Fiber	3g
Sugar	2g
Protein	14g

¾ cup Tessemae's Creamy Ranch Dressing

2 cups shredded barbecue chicken (see sidebar)

1½ cups coleslaw

¾ cup fire-roasted corn kernels

6 tablespoons minced red onion

12 cups chopped romaine lettuce

1. Layer 2 tablespoons dressing, ⅓ cup chicken, ¼ cup coleslaw, 2 tablespoons corn, 1 tablespoon onion, and 2 cups lettuce each into six wide-mouth quart-sized Mason jars.
2. Cover and store in refrigerator until ready to eat, up to 1 week. When ready to serve, shake vigorously.

EASY BULK BARBECUE CHICKEN

Making a huge batch of shredded barbecue chicken could not be easier, so work it into your meal prep rotation as much as you can. Combine 3 pounds of boneless, skinless chicken breasts with 1½ cups (around 12 ounces) no-sugar-added barbecue sauce in a slow cooker, cover, and cook on low for 6–8 hours or until chicken shreds easily with a fork. When it's done, shred it with two forks, stir it around in the barbecue sauce, and then use in your recipes or freeze for later, up to 3 months.

Thai Peanut Salad

SERVES 6

Per Serving:

Calories	378
Fat	19g
Sodium	537mg
Carbohydrates	12g
Fiber	6g
Sugar	3g
Protein	39g

If you have some extra room in your carb allowance, you can add some cooked rice noodles or soba noodles to this salad for a delicious contrast in texture.

FOR SALAD

1 (16-ounce) package coleslaw mix

3 cups shredded cooked boneless, skinless chicken breasts

1 large red pepper, seeded and finely diced

½ cup chopped peanuts

3 medium scallions, chopped

2 tablespoons chopped Thai basil

½ teaspoon sea salt

¼ teaspoon ground black pepper

FOR SAUCE

6 tablespoons no-sugar-added creamy peanut butter

2 tablespoons coconut aminos

2 tablespoons pulp-free orange juice

1 tablespoon lime juice

1 tablespoon ChocZero Maple-Flavored Syrup

1 tablespoon sriracha

1 teaspoon toasted sesame oil

2 cloves garlic, peeled and minced

2 teaspoons seeded minced jalapeño

1 teaspoon grated fresh ginger

1. To make Salad: Add all ingredients to a large bowl and mix well. Divide evenly into six airtight containers.
2. To make Sauce: Whisk all ingredients in a small bowl until smooth. Divide evenly into six small dressing containers. Place small containers in Salad containers, cover, and store in refrigerator until ready to eat, up to 1 week.
3. When ready to serve, pour Sauce over Salad and shake to coat.

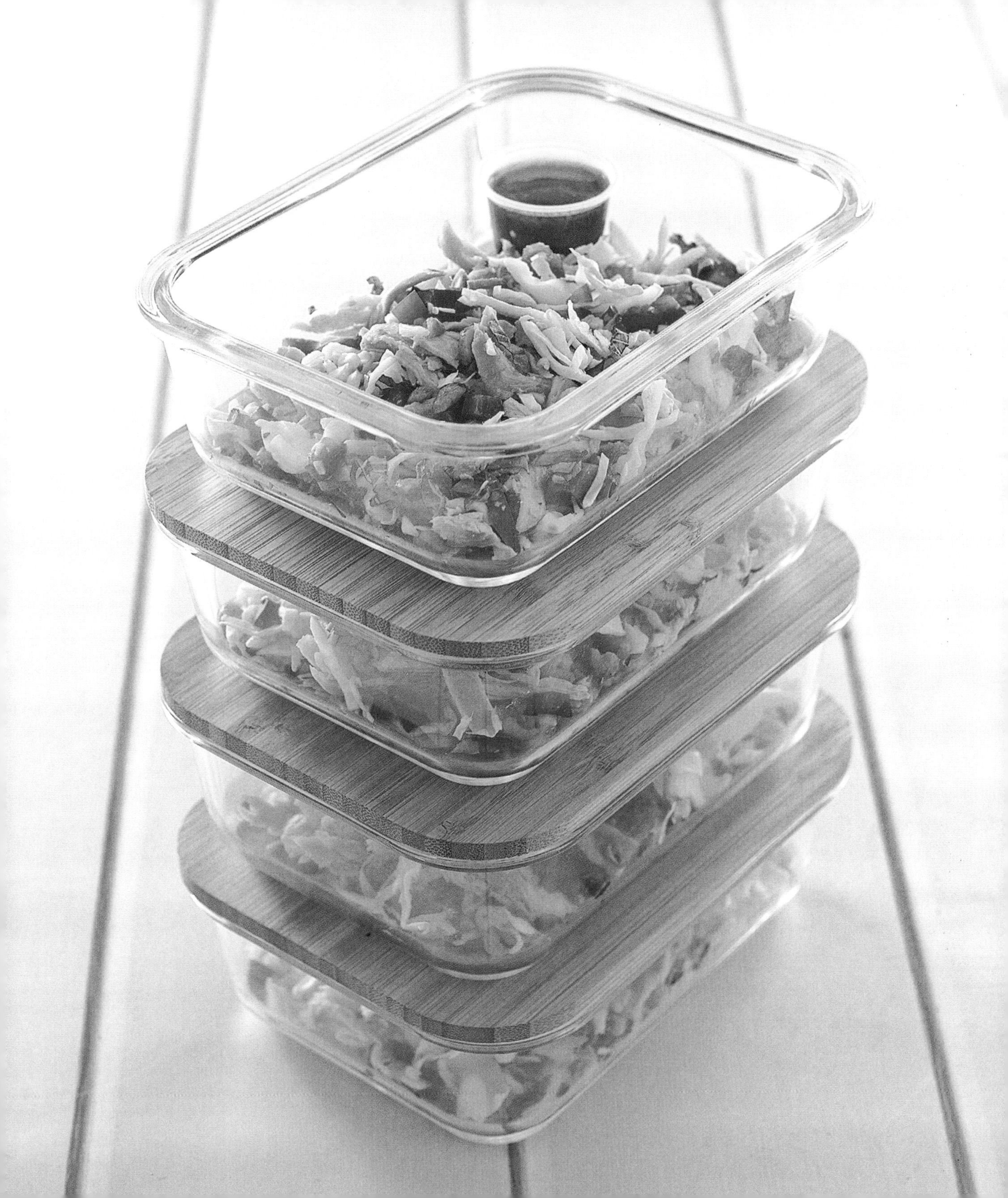

Salmon Caesar Salad

SERVES 6

Per Serving:

Calories	293
Fat	16g
Sodium	356mg
Carbohydrates	12g
Fiber	4g
Sugar	2g
Protein	26g

ROASTING YOUR CHICKPEAS

Thanks to their beautiful macronutrient profile—½ cup contains 6 grams of fat, 60 grams of carbohydrates, and 19.5 grams of protein—chickpeas should be a staple in any macro diet. Canned chickpeas are already cooked, so you can eat them after rinsing, but roasting them with a little bit of oil and some spices turns them into something special. For basic roasted chickpeas, toss a can of chickpeas (drained and rinsed) with a teaspoon of olive oil and a sprinkle of salt, spread them out on a baking sheet, and roast at 400°F for 25 minutes.

Because this recipe is so basic, it's easy to customize. Instead of salmon, you can use cooked chicken, canned tuna, or a vegetarian source of protein like beans, chickpeas, or tofu.

¾ cup Tessemae's Creamy Caesar Dressing
3 (6-ounce) cans wild salmon, drained
6 teaspoons grated Parmesan cheese
12 cups chopped romaine lettuce
¾ cup roasted chickpeas

1. Layer 2 tablespoons dressing, ½ can salmon, 1 teaspoon Parmesan, 2 cups lettuce, and 2 tablespoons chickpeas in each of six wide-mouth quart-sized Mason jars.
2. Cover and store in refrigerator until ready to eat, up to 1 week. When ready to serve, shake vigorously.

Greek Shrimp Salad

Raw zoodles, or zucchini noodles, have a nice crunch that goes away when you cook them. This Greek Shrimp Salad keeps the noodles raw to add some texture when you're ready to eat it. If you want even more crunch, and some protein, you can add a handful of nuts or seeds to the jars.

SERVES 6

Per Serving:

Calories	351
Fat	30g
Sodium	988mg
Carbohydrates	5g
Fiber	1g
Sugar	3g
Protein	17g

6 tablespoons extra-virgin olive oil

6 tablespoons lemon juice

1 tablespoon dried oregano

3⁄4 teaspoon sea salt

3⁄4 teaspoon ground black pepper

1½ cups cooked peeled deveined small shrimp

3⁄4 cup chopped red onion

3⁄4 cup chopped kalamata olives

3⁄4 cup crumbled feta cheese

3 medium zucchini, spiralized

1. Whisk together oil, lemon juice, oregano, salt, and pepper in a small bowl. Add 2 tablespoons dressing each to six quart-sized Mason jars.
2. Layer ¼ cup shrimp, 2 tablespoons onion, 2 tablespoons olives, 2 tablespoons feta, and zoodles from ½ zucchini in each jar.
3. Cover and store in refrigerator until ready to eat, up to 1 week. When ready to serve, shake vigorously.

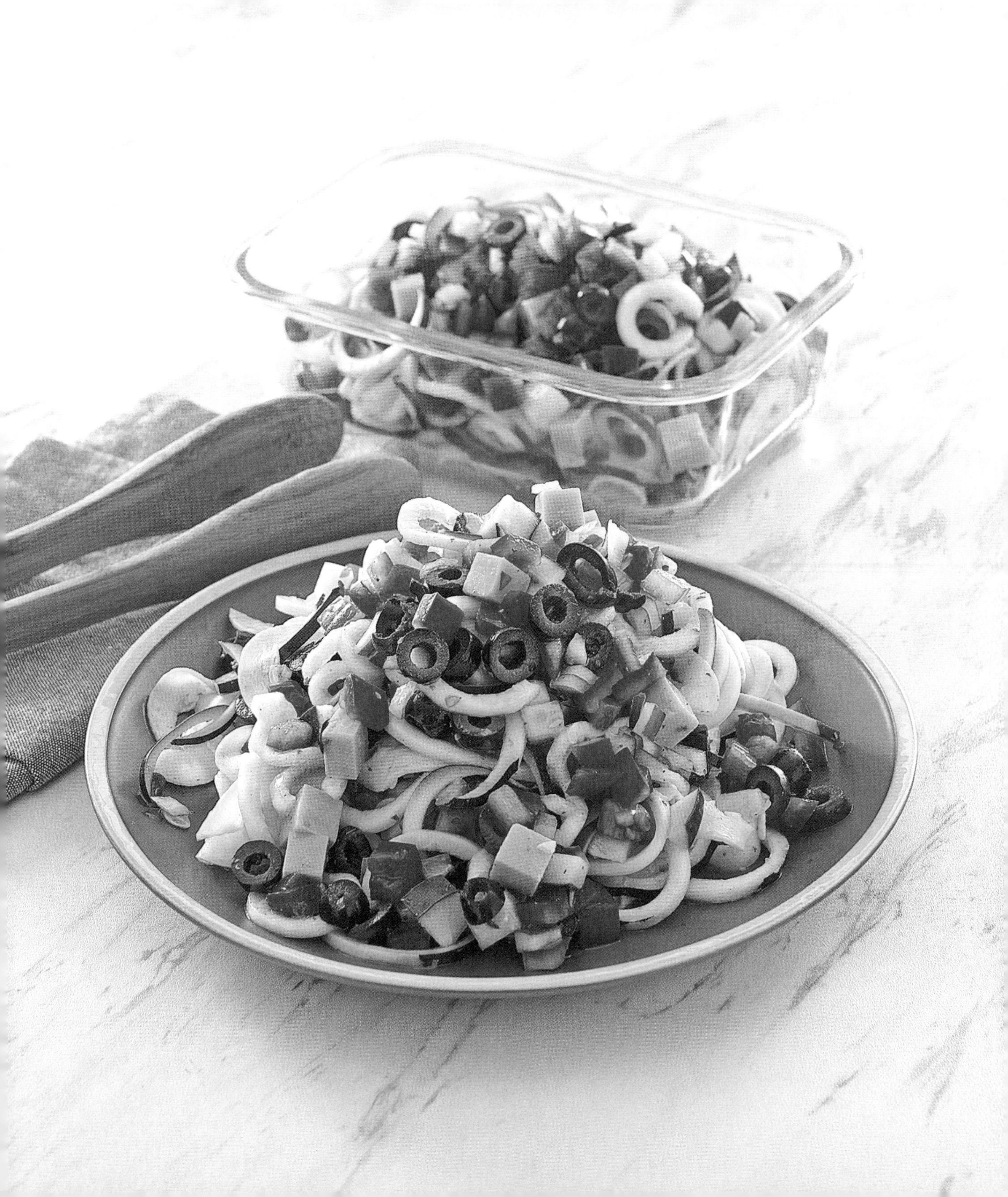

Zoodle Pasta Salad

When meal prepping, make sure you're storing the dressing and zoodles separately. Otherwise, the zoodles will get a bit soggy as they sit in the refrigerator. They'll still be edible, but they'll be missing that little crunch that makes this pasta salad so satisfying.

SERVES 6

Per Serving:

Calories	203
Fat	13g
Sodium	345mg
Carbohydrates	10g
Fiber	3g
Sugar	7g
Protein	11g

2 large zucchini, spiralized

1 medium yellow squash, spiralized

3 medium Roma tomatoes, diced

2 medium red bell peppers, seeded and diced

1 medium red onion, finely diced

1 large cucumber, diced

1 (6-ounce) can olives, drained and sliced

1 (8-ounce) block sharp Cheddar cheese, cut into 1⁄4" cubes

3⁄4 cup Tessemae's Classic Greek Dressing and Marinade

1. Combine all ingredients, except dressing, in a large bowl. Divide evenly into six airtight containers.
2. Pour 2 tablespoons dressing into each of six small containers. Place small containers in salad containers, cover, and refrigerate until ready to eat, up to 1 week.
3. When ready to serve, add dressing to salad and shake to coat.

Chopped Bean and Corn Salad

SERVES 6

Per Serving:

Calories	381
Fat	18g
Sodium	310mg
Carbohydrates	44g
Fiber	9g
Sugar	8g
Protein	10g

This vegan-friendly salad comes together in minutes. There's no cooking involved—all you have to do is open a couple cans, chop some vegetables, and you have a protein- and fiber-packed meal for days.

1 (15-ounce) can black beans, drained and rinsed
1 (15-ounce) can chickpeas, drained and rinsed
1 (12-ounce) can sweet corn kernels, drained
½ cup chopped English cucumber
½ cup finely chopped red onion
¼ cup chopped fresh cilantro
1 large ripe avocado, pitted, peeled, and chopped
1 large red bell pepper, seeded and finely chopped
½ cup cooked white rice
¾ cup Tessemae's Honey Poppyseed Dressing and Marinade

1. Combine all ingredients, except dressing, in a large bowl and mix well. Pour dressing on top and toss to coat.
2. Divide evenly into six airtight containers. Cover and store in refrigerator until ready to eat, up to 1 week. Serve cold.

High-Protein Lentil Salad

Thanks to the combination of brown lentils and shredded chicken, this salad is absolutely packed with protein. If it's too much to fit into your daily macros, you can reduce the amount of either or both, or just use one instead of the combination.

SERVES 6

Per Serving:

Calories	252
Fat	11g
Sodium	316mg
Carbohydrates	16g
Fiber	10g
Sugar	2g
Protein	22g

FOR SALAD

2 cups cooked brown lentils
1 cup shredded cooked boneless, skinless chicken breasts
1 large cucumber, seeded and diced
⅓ cup chopped sun-dried tomatoes
½ cup diced red bell pepper
¼ cup peeled shredded carrot
¼ cup sliced green olives
3 tablespoons chopped fresh basil

FOR DRESSING

3 tablespoons extra-virgin olive oil
2 tablespoons apple cider vinegar
1 tablespoon lemon juice
1 tablespoon ChocZero Maple-Flavored Syrup
2 tablespoons tahini
½ teaspoon dried oregano
½ teaspoon sea salt
¼ teaspoon ground black pepper

1. To make Salad: Combine all ingredients in a large bowl.
2. To make Dressing: Whisk all ingredients in a small bowl until smooth. Pour Dressing over Salad and toss to coat.
3. Divide into six airtight containers. Cover and store in refrigerator until ready to eat, up to 1 week. Serve cold.

GETTING THE RIGHT AMOUNT OF PROTEIN

When it comes to protein, a lot of people think more is better, but that's not always the case. You should aim for 0.8 to 1 gram of protein per kilogram of body weight if you have normal activity levels. If you lift heavy weights regularly, you can bump it up to 1.2 to 1.4 grams per kilogram. High-protein foods, like lentils and chicken, will help you meet your protein needs a lot more easily than you may realize.

CHAPTER 4

Soups, Stews, and Chili

Instant Pot® Turkey Chili

SERVES 6

Per Serving:

Calories	391
Fat	10g
Sodium	736mg
Carbohydrates	43g
Fiber	11g
Sugar	18g
Protein	32g

Because tomato-based meals like chili get even tastier after spending a few days in the refrigerator, they're an excellent option for meal prepping. And thanks to the use of an Instant Pot®, this version comes together in no time. If you want to cut the carbs a bit, you can omit the beans.

2 teaspoons extra-virgin olive oil
2 cloves garlic, peeled and minced
1 large yellow onion, peeled and diced
2 medium red bell peppers, seeded and diced
1½ pounds 90% lean ground turkey
1 tablespoon chili powder
1 tablespoon paprika
1 tablespoon garlic powder
1½ teaspoons ground cumin
1½ teaspoons onion powder
½ teaspoon sea salt
½ teaspoon ground black pepper
1 (14-ounce) can petite-diced tomatoes, including juice
1 (15-ounce) can no-sugar-added tomato sauce
1 (15-ounce) can red kidney beans, drained and rinsed

1. Set to Sauté function and heat up oil. Add garlic, onion, and peppers and cook, stirring occasionally, until softened, about 5 minutes. Add remaining ingredients to pot and stir well to combine.
2. Close lid, choose Soup setting, and set time for 30 minutes. When time is up, allow pressure to release naturally. Open lid and allow chili to cool 1 hour.
3. Divide chili evenly into six airtight containers. Store in refrigerator up to 1 week, or in freezer up to 3 months, until ready to eat.
4. To serve, transfer to a saucepan and cook over medium heat 5 minutes or until heated through.

Creamy Taco Soup

If you don't have cooked chicken breast on hand and you want to make this recipe even easier, grab a rotisserie chicken from the store and use the meat from that. Just make sure to read the nutrition facts and choose one that doesn't have added ingredients that negatively affect your macros.

SERVES 6

Per Serving:

Calories	350
Fat	4g
Sodium	665mg
Carbohydrates	44g
Fiber	14g
Sugar	4g
Protein	34g

1 (15-ounce) can black beans, drained and rinsed
1 (15-ounce) can pinto beans, drained and rinsed
1 (14.5-ounce) can petite-diced tomatoes, including juice
1½ cups shredded cooked boneless, skinless chicken breast
1 (15-ounce) can refried beans
1 (14-ounce) can chicken broth
1 (4-ounce) can green chiles, including juice
1 (1.3-ounce) packet Siete Taco Seasoning

1. Combine all ingredients in a slow cooker. Stir until everything is smooth.
2. Cover and cook on low 3 hours. Turn off slow cooker and allow to cool 1 hour.
3. Divide soup evenly into six airtight containers. Store in refrigerator up to 1 week, or in freezer up to 3 months, until ready to serve.
4. To serve, transfer to a saucepan and cook over medium heat 5 minutes, or microwave 1 minute, or until heated through.

Paleo Pumpkin Chili

SERVES 6

Per Serving:

Calories	297
Fat	16g
Sodium	680mg
Carbohydrates	20g
Fiber	4g
Sugar	8g
Protein	18g

FRESH PUMPKIN PURÉE

If you prefer to make your own pumpkin purée rather than using the canned kind, it's really easy to do. Cut a small (but not baby) pumpkin in half, put it face-down on a parchment paper-lined baking sheet, and roast at 350°F for 45 minutes. Let it cool down a little, scoop the flesh out of the skin, and blend in a food processor until smooth. Use it right away or freeze for later.

If you want to stock your freezer with extra meals, you can easily double or triple this recipe, freeze what you won't eat in a week, and save the rest for later. If you freeze your soups and chilis in individual portion sizes, you can heat each one up right in the microwave when you need a quick meal.

2 tablespoons chili powder

2 teaspoons ground cumin

1 teaspoon unsweetened cocoa powder

1 teaspoon dried oregano

1 teaspoon salt

½ teaspoon ground cinnamon

¼ teaspoon ground allspice

2 tablespoons extra-virgin olive oil

1 small white onion, peeled and finely diced

2 cloves garlic, peeled and minced

1 pound 85% lean grass-fed ground beef

2 medium sweet potatoes, peeled and diced

1 (15-ounce) can pumpkin purée

1 (14.5-ounce) can fire-roasted diced tomatoes, including juice

2 cups beef broth

1. Mix chili powder, cumin, cocoa powder, oregano, salt, cinnamon, and allspice in a small bowl. Set aside.
2. Heat oil in a large stockpot or Dutch oven over medium heat. Add onion and garlic and cook until translucent, about 5 minutes. Add beef and cook until no longer pink, about 8 minutes. Add spice mixture and stir until incorporated.
3. Add remaining ingredients and stir until combined. Simmer over low heat 2 hours, stirring occasionally. Remove from heat and allow to cool 1 hour.
4. Divide evenly into six airtight containers. Store in refrigerator up to 1 week, or in freezer up to 3 months, until ready to eat.
5. To serve, transfer to a saucepan and cook over medium heat 5 minutes, or microwave 1 minute, or until heated through.

Tomato and Red Pepper Soup

If you want to reduce the fat content of this soup, you can swap out the coconut milk and use chicken broth or vegetable broth instead. It will be a little less creamy, but every bit as delicious.

SERVES 6

Per Serving:

Calories	259
Fat	13g
Sodium	476mg
Carbohydrates	30g
Fiber	10g
Sugar	14g
Protein	6g

3 large red bell peppers

1 tablespoon extra-virgin olive oil

1 medium yellow onion, peeled and chopped

2 medium carrots, peeled and diced

2 medium stalks celery, diced

4 cloves garlic, peeled and minced

1 (28-ounce) can crushed tomatoes

1 (15-ounce) can peeled tomatoes, including juice

2 (6-ounce) cans tomato paste

2 (14-ounce) cans light coconut milk

2 tablespoons dried dill

1½ teaspoons dried basil

1 teaspoon sea salt

½ teaspoon ground black pepper

¼ teaspoon red pepper flakes

1. Preheat oven to 500°F. Line a baking sheet with aluminum foil.
2. Place bell peppers on prepared baking sheet and roast 15 minutes or until skin is charred. Wrap aluminum foil around each pepper and allow to steam inside foil packet 10 minutes.
3. While peppers are steaming, heat oil in a large stockpot or Dutch oven over medium-high heat. Add onion and cook 4 minutes. Add carrots and celery and cook until carrots start to soften, about 5 minutes. Stir in garlic and cook 1 more minute.
4. Add remaining ingredients to pot and stir to combine. Reduce heat to low.
5. Carefully remove peppers from foil and remove skin, seeds, and stems. Roughly chop peppers and add to soup. Stir to combine.
6. Use an immersion blender to purée soup, or transfer to a blender in batches and blend until smooth, then return to pot.
7. Let soup simmer 1 hour, then remove from heat and allow to cool 1 hour.
8. Divide evenly into six airtight containers. Store in refrigerator up to 1 week, or in freezer, up to 3 months, until ready to eat.
9. To serve, transfer to a saucepan and cook over medium heat 5 minutes, or microwave 1 minute, or until heated through.

Pumpkin and Bacon Soup

SERVES 6

Per Serving:

Calories	98
Fat	3g
Sodium	853mg
Carbohydrates	11g
Fiber	2g
Sugar	5g
Protein	7g

If you have some fat macros to spare and you want to make this soup extra creamy, you can stir in a tablespoon or two of half-and-half before eating (but after reheating so the cream doesn't curdle).

6 slices no-sugar-added bacon, roughly chopped
1 small white onion, peeled and finely minced
2 cloves garlic, peeled and minced
1 (15-ounce) can pumpkin purée
1 teaspoon sea salt
½ teaspoon ground black pepper
8 cups chicken broth

1. Cook bacon in a large stockpot or Dutch oven over medium-high heat 5 minutes. Reduce heat to medium, add onion and garlic, and cook another 2 minutes or until bacon is crispy. Drain bacon fat.
2. Add remaining ingredients to pot and stir well to combine. Reduce heat to low and let simmer 1 hour. Remove from heat and allow to cool 1 hour.
3. Divide evenly into six airtight containers. Store in refrigerator up to 1 week, or in freezer up to 3 months, until ready to eat.
4. To serve, transfer to a saucepan and cook over medium heat 5 minutes, or microwave 1 minute, or until heated through.

Creamy Quinoa Soup

Quinoa adds a nice texture and earthy taste to this soup, but if you prefer rice (and it fits into your macros better) you can use any type in its place. You may need to simmer for a bit longer, however, especially if you're using brown rice.

SERVES 6

Per Serving:

Calories	396
Fat	11g
Sodium	854mg
Carbohydrates	55g
Fiber	12g
Sugar	12g
Protein	18g

1 tablespoon extra-virgin olive oil
2 large shallots, peeled and minced
2 large carrots, peeled and diced
1 medium stalk celery, diced
5 cloves garlic, peeled and minced
½ teaspoon sea salt
¼ teaspoon ground black pepper
4 cups chicken broth
1 (15-ounce) can chickpeas, drained and rinsed
1 (15-ounce) can tomato sauce
1 (14.5-ounce) can fire-roasted tomatoes, including juice
4 cups chopped kale
1¼ cups sprouted quinoa, rinsed
1 tablespoon Italian seasoning
¼ cup organic light cream

1. Heat oil in a large stockpot or Dutch oven. Add shallot, carrots, and celery and cook until carrots start to soften, about 5 minutes. Add garlic and cook another 2 minutes. Sprinkle salt and pepper over vegetable mixture and stir.
2. Add remaining ingredients, except cream, and stir until combined. Reduce heat to medium-low and simmer 30 minutes. Remove from heat and stir in cream. Allow to cool 1 hour.
3. Divide evenly into six airtight containers. Store in refrigerator up to 1 week, or in freezer up to 3 months, until ready to eat.
4. To serve, transfer to a saucepan and cook over medium heat 5 minutes, or microwave 1 minute, or until heated through.

GIVE QUINOA AN EXTRA RINSE

Quinoa has a natural coating on it, called saponin, that can make it taste bitter or soapy if not removed. Thoroughly rinsing quinoa before you cook it removes most of the saponin, giving you a better result. If you buy quinoa that's labeled as "pre-rinsed," you can skip this step.

Broccoli Cheese Soup

SERVES 6

Per Serving:

Calories	285
Fat	17g
Sodium	685mg
Carbohydrates	17g
Fiber	1g
Sugar	1g
Protein	14g

The potatoes in this soup help thicken it up a bit, but if you're watching your carb intake or you've reached your carb quota for the week, you can omit them. The soup will still be delicious.

1 tablespoon extra-virgin olive oil
2 large carrots, peeled and diced
2 medium stalks celery, diced
1 medium yellow onion, peeled and diced
4 cloves garlic, peeled and minced
4 cups broccoli florets
2 cups diced peeled yellow potatoes
1 teaspoon sea salt
½ teaspoon ground black pepper
3 cups chicken broth
½ cup organic light cream
1½ cups shredded Cheddar cheese

1. Set pressure cooker to Sauté function and heat up oil. Add carrots and celery and cook 5 minutes. Add onion and cook another 4 minutes. Stir in garlic and cook 1 more minute.
2. Add broccoli, potatoes, salt, pepper, and broth and stir. Close pressure cooker lid, choose high pressure, and set time for 4 minutes. When time is up, release pressure manually.
3. Carefully open lid and scoop out 1 cup broccoli with tongs or a slotted spoon. Set aside.
4. Stir in cream, then purée soup with an immersion blender. Stir in cheese until cheese is melted and soup is smooth. Stir in reserved broccoli.
5. Allow to cool 1 hour, then divide evenly into six airtight containers. Store in refrigerator up to 1 week, or in freezer up to 3 months, until ready to eat.
6. To serve, transfer to a saucepan and cook over medium heat 5 minutes, or microwave 1 minute, or until heated through.

Loaded Baked Potato Soup

If you want to cut the carbs in this recipe, you can use half potatoes and half turnips, or completely replace the potatoes with turnips, which have a similar taste and texture. For comparison, 1 cup of diced turnips contains 8 grams of carbs, while a cup of diced potatoes has 26 grams—and you'll barely even notice the difference in the finished soup!

SERVES 6

Per Serving:

Calories	251
Fat	7g
Sodium	384mg
Carbohydrates	34g
Fiber	3g
Sugar	6g
Protein	13g

4 slices no-sugar-added bacon, chopped

½ cup diced yellow onion

½ cup peeled diced carrots

¼ cup diced celery

4 cups peeled diced russet potatoes

4 cups chicken broth

1 teaspoon garlic powder

½ teaspoon sea salt

½ teaspoon ground black pepper

2 cups 2% organic milk

2 ounces cream cheese

1. Add bacon to a medium skillet and cook over medium heat 2 minutes. Add onion, carrots, and celery and continue to cook until carrots start to soften, about 6 minutes. Transfer to slow cooker.
2. Add potatoes, broth, garlic powder, salt, and pepper to slow cooker, cover, and cook 6 hours on high.
3. Add milk and cream cheese, cover, and cook another 30 minutes, stirring occasionally to melt cream cheese.
4. Using a slotted spoon, scoop out half of potatoes and transfer to a blender or food processor. Process until puréed, about 1 minute. Pour back into slow cooker and stir to combine. Turn off slow cooker and allow to cool 1 hour.
5. Divide evenly into six airtight containers. Store in refrigerator up to 1 week or in freezer, up to 3 months, until ready to eat.
6. To serve, transfer to a saucepan and cook over medium heat 5 minutes, or microwave 1 minute, or until heated through.

HOW TO PREP TURNIPS

If you've never used turnips before, it may feel intimidating, but prepping them is just as easy as preparing potatoes. Wash the turnips thoroughly, then cut off the green tops. Use a vegetable peeler to remove the skin, then cut the turnip into cubes. It takes about 10 minutes to cook turnips in hot liquid.

Buffalo Chicken Soup with Blue Cheese Crumbles

SERVES 6

Per Serving:

Calories	398
Fat	24g
Sodium	700mg
Carbohydrates	13g
Fiber	1g
Sugar	3g
Protein	26g

The blue cheese crumbles in this recipe aren't added until after the soup is reheated. To make meal prep simpler, you can add 1 table-spoon of blue cheese to a small snack bag and tape it to each container before storing in the refrigerator. That way, you have the cheese portioned and ready to go when it comes time to eat the soup. Feel free to add chopped cilantro as a garnish before serving.

1 tablespoon unsalted grass-fed butter
1 small yellow onion, peeled and diced
2 medium stalks celery, finely diced
3 ounces cream cheese
½ cup organic light cream
4 cups chicken broth
⅓ cup Noble Made Medium Buffalo Sauce
3 cups shredded cooked boneless, skinless chicken breasts
1 cup shredded Cheddar cheese
½ cup shredded Colby Jack cheese
6 tablespoons crumbled blue cheese

1. Heat butter in a large stockpot or Dutch oven over medium-high heat. Add onion and celery and cook 5 minutes or until celery starts to soften.
2. Reduce heat to low and add cream cheese and cream. Stir until cream cheese is melted and mixture is smooth. Stir in broth and buffalo sauce. Add chicken and simmer 10 minutes.
3. Add Cheddar and Colby Jack in small batches, stirring after each batch until cheese melts and soup is smooth. Remove from heat and allow to cool 1 hour.
4. Divide evenly into six airtight containers. Store in refrigerator up to 1 week or in freezer up to 3 months, until ready to eat.
5. To serve, transfer to a saucepan and cook over medium heat 5 minutes, or microwave 1 minute, or until heated through. Serve with 1 tablespoon blue cheese crumbles on top.

CELLULOSE IN SHREDDED CHEESE

Most packaged shredded cheese contains a carbohydrate filler called cellulose that acts as an anti-caking agent, or a substance that prevents the cheese from clumping together. While cellulose is a natural component found in vegetables, the type of cellulose in shredded cheese is highly processed and interferes with the way the cheese melts, leaving you with a grainy finished dish. Whenever you can, try to shred cheese from a block yourself.

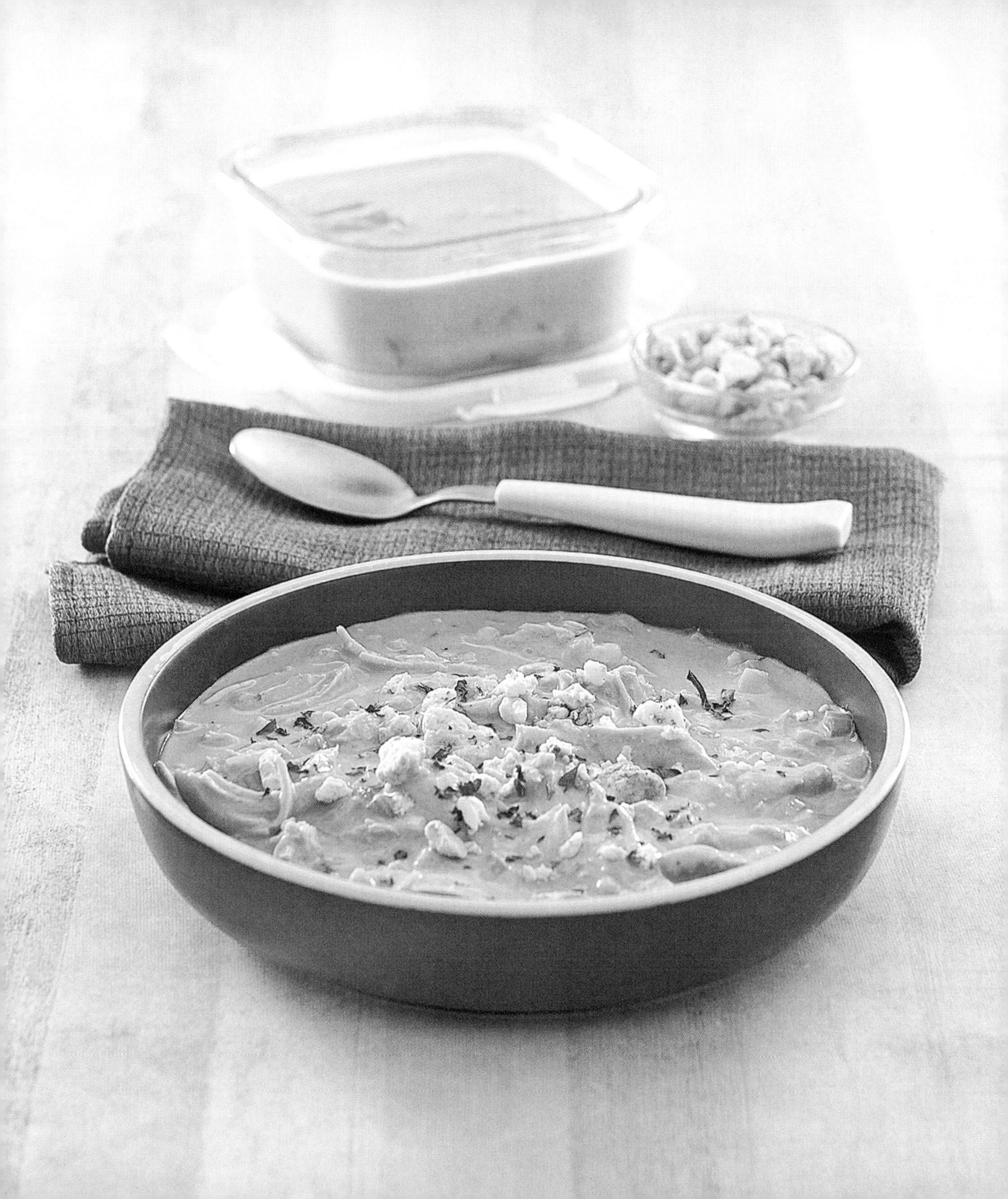

Sweet Potato and Carrot Soup

SERVES 6

Per Serving:

Calories	143
Fat	8g
Sodium	578mg
Carbohydrates	15g
Fiber	1g
Sugar	3g
Protein	3g

If you don't have an immersion blender, you can transfer portions of the soup to a regular blender and carefully blend it in batches. Be sure to remove the center cap of the blender lid and hold a towel over the hole to allow steam to escape, or else you risk an explosion of hot liquid!

2 tablespoons extra-virgin olive oil
2 cloves garlic, peeled and minced
1 small yellow onion, peeled and minced
1 tablespoon grated fresh ginger
4 cups chicken broth
1 cup peeled sliced carrots
1 cup peeled cubed sweet potatoes
½ teaspoon ground cumin
½ teaspoon sea salt
½ cup organic half-and-half

1. Heat oil in a large stockpot or Dutch oven over medium heat. Add garlic, onion, and ginger and cook 3 minutes.
2. Add remaining ingredients, except half-and-half, and stir. Bring to a boil over high heat, reduce heat to low, and simmer 45 minutes or until sweet potatoes are tender.
3. Remove from heat and use an immersion blender to purée soup. Allow to cool 20 minutes, then stir in half-and-half.
4. Divide evenly into six airtight containers. Store in refrigerator up to 1 week, or in freezer up to 3 months, until ready to eat.
5. To serve, transfer to a saucepan and cook over medium heat 5 minutes, or microwave 1 minute, or until heated through.

Cheddar Cauliflower Soup

If you want to make this recipe vegan-friendly, simply replace the chicken broth with vegetable broth. And if you want to increase the protein, you can add some shredded cooked chicken in after you purée the soup.

SERVES 6

Per Serving:

Calories	104
Fat	4g
Sodium	526mg
Carbohydrates	11g
Fiber	3g
Sugar	3g
Protein	6g

1 large head cauliflower, chopped
3 medium stalks celery, chopped
2 cloves garlic, peeled and minced
1 large sweet onion, peeled and chopped
2 teaspoons ground cumin
½ teaspoon ground black pepper
4½ cups chicken broth
½ cup shredded Cheddar cheese

1. Combine all ingredients, except cheese, in a large stockpot or Dutch oven. Bring to a boil over high heat, then reduce heat to low and simmer 10 minutes or until cauliflower is tender.
2. Use an immersion blender to purée soup. Simmer another 20 minutes. Remove from heat and stir in cheese until it melts. Allow to cool 1 hour.
3. Divide evenly into six airtight containers. Store in refrigerator up to 1 week or in freezer up to 3 months, until ready to eat.
4. To serve, transfer to a saucepan and cook over medium heat 5 minutes, or microwave 1 minute, or until heated through.

Beef and Mushroom Stew

SERVES 6

Per Serving:	
Calories	245
Fat	10g
Sodium	545mg
Carbohydrates	2g
Fiber	2g
Sugar	1g
Protein	37g

WHAT IS ARROWROOT POWDER?

Arrowroot is a root vegetable that's often dried and transformed into gluten-free powder. It has no taste and is most commonly used as a thickener in place of cornstarch. Unlike cornstarch, arrowroot powder is processed naturally and without high heat, so the powder stays free of unwanted chemicals and artificial ingredients and retains most of its nutrients.

If you don't have arrowroot powder, you can use cornstarch in its place. Simply use 1 teaspoon of cornstarch and 1 teaspoon of water to make the slurry.

- 2 pounds chuck stew meat, cut into 1" cubes
- 2 tablespoons Bob's Red Mill Paleo Baking Flour
- 1 tablespoon unsalted grass-fed butter
- 2 large shallots, peeled and minced
- 1½ pounds sliced shiitake mushrooms
- 2 cups beef broth, divided
- 2 tablespoons tomato paste
- 1 teaspoon Trader Joe's Multipurpose Umami Seasoning Blend
- 1 teaspoon dried rosemary
- 1 teaspoon sea salt
- ½ teaspoon ground black pepper
- ½ teaspoon garlic powder
- ½ teaspoon onion powder
- 2 bay leaves
- 2 teaspoons arrowroot powder
- 2 teaspoons water

1. Add beef to a large zip-top bag. Sprinkle flour into bag and shake to coat.
2. Heat butter in a large stockpot or Dutch oven over medium-high heat. Add beef to pot and cook 2 minutes on each side or until all sides are browned. Transfer with a slotted spoon to a plate.
3. Add shallot and mushrooms to pot and cook until mushrooms start to soften, about 5 minutes. Pour in ¼ cup broth and scrape bottom of Dutch oven to release browned bits.
4. Stir in remaining 1¾ cups broth and remaining ingredients, except arrowroot and water. Return browned beef to Dutch oven, stir, and bring to a boil. Reduce heat to low and simmer 1½ hours or until beef is cooked through and tender.
5. Whisk arrowroot and water in a small bowl until smooth. Add to beef stew and stir to mix. Simmer another 30 minutes. Remove from heat and allow to cool 1 hour.
6. Divide evenly into six airtight containers. Store in refrigerator up to 1 week, or in freezer up to 3 months, until ready to eat.
7. To serve, transfer to a saucepan and cook over medium heat 5 minutes, or microwave 1 minute, or until heated through.

Coconut Curry Lentil Soup

Make sure you're using light coconut milk for this recipe. If you get the full-fat version, it will significantly change the fat content of each serving. If you can't find light coconut milk, you can mix equal parts of the full-fat version with filtered water.

SERVES 6

Per Serving:

Calories	263
Fat	7g
Sodium	579mg
Carbohydrates	35g
Fiber	4g
Sugar	7g
Protein	15g

- 2 teaspoons toasted sesame oil
- 1 teaspoon grated fresh ginger
- 3 cloves garlic, peeled and minced
- 2 tablespoons red curry paste
- ¼ cup minced red onion
- ½ teaspoon sea salt
- ½ teaspoon ground black pepper
- 1 tablespoon coconut aminos
- 1½ cups dried red lentils, rinsed
- 1 (14-ounce) can light coconut milk
- 5 cups no-sugar-added vegetable broth
- 1 tablespoon fresh lime juice
- 1 tablespoon sriracha
- 2 cups chopped kale

1. Heat oil in a large skillet over medium-high heat. Add ginger, garlic, and curry paste and stir to mix. Cook 1 minute. Stir in onion, salt, pepper, and coconut aminos and cook another 5 minutes or until translucent.
2. Stir in lentils, coconut milk, and broth. Bring to a boil, reduce heat to low, and simmer 45 minutes, stirring occasionally. Stir in lime juice, sriracha, and kale and simmer another 3 minutes. Remove from heat and allow to cool 1 hour.
3. Divide evenly into six airtight containers. Cover and store in refrigerator up to 1 week, or in freezer up to 3 months, until ready to eat.
4. To serve, transfer to a saucepan and cook over medium heat 5 minutes, or microwave 1 minute, or until heated through.

SHAKE YOUR COCONUT MILK

Coconut milk that comes in a can is a lot different than the boxed or bottled coconut milk you may be used to. Because canned coconut milk has fewer added ingredients (some brands don't have any), when you open it, you might notice that there's a thick layer on top and a liquid layer on bottom. This is perfectly normal—it's the fat separating from the water. You can either shake the coconut milk vigorously to mix it or pulse it a couple times in a food processor before using.

Spicy Black Bean Soup

SERVES 6

Per Serving:

Calories	208
Fat	4g
Sodium	566mg
Carbohydrates	32g
Fiber	11g
Sugar	7g
Protein	11g

This soup packs some heat, but if you want to dial it down, you can omit the cayenne pepper and use regular diced tomatoes in place of the fire-roasted without significantly changing the macros.

1 tablespoon extra-virgin olive oil

1 medium white onion, peeled and chopped

2 cloves garlic, peeled and minced

1 medium stalk celery, chopped

1 medium carrot, peeled and chopped

1 tablespoon chili powder

1 teaspoon ground cumin

½ teaspoon sea salt

½ teaspoon ground black pepper

¼ teaspoon cayenne pepper

4 cups chicken broth

2 (15-ounce) cans black beans, drained and rinsed, divided

1 (14.5-ounce) can fire-roasted diced tomatoes, drained

1. Heat oil in a large stockpot or Dutch oven over medium heat. Add onion and garlic and cook 3 minutes or until onion starts to become translucent. Add celery and carrot and cook another 5 minutes or until carrot starts to become tender. Stir in chili powder, cumin, salt, black pepper, and cayenne pepper.
2. Add broth and 1 can beans. Bring to a boil, then reduce heat to low.
3. Combine remaining beans and tomatoes in a food processor and process 30 seconds or until smooth. Stir purée into soup. Cover and simmer 30 minutes. Remove from heat and allow to cool 1 hour.
4. Divide evenly into six airtight containers. Store in refrigerator up to 1 week, or in freezer up to 3 months, until ready to eat.
5. To serve, transfer to a saucepan and cook over medium heat 5 minutes, or microwave 1 minute, or until heated through.

Chicken and Kale Stew

This soup is simple, hearty, and easily adaptable. If you want to cut carbs, you can omit the potatoes or the beans (or cut back on both). You can also use whatever combination of vegetables works for your macros and your taste buds.

SERVES 6

Per Serving:

Calories	224
Fat	4g
Sodium	560mg
Carbohydrates	20g
Fiber	6g
Sugar	3g
Protein	25g

1 tablespoon extra-virgin olive oil

1 cup chopped leeks

1 large carrot, peeled and finely diced

3 cloves garlic, peeled and minced

3 (4-ounce) boneless, skinless chicken breasts, cut into 1" cubes

6 cups chicken broth

1 cup peeled diced yellow potatoes

6 cups chopped kale

1 (15-ounce) can cannellini beans, drained and rinsed

1 teaspoon sea salt

½ teaspoon ground black pepper

½ teaspoon dried thyme

2 tablespoons Dijon mustard

1. Heat oil in a large stockpot or Dutch oven over medium heat. Add leeks and carrot and cook 5 minutes or until starting to soften. Add garlic and cook 1 more minute.
2. Add chicken and cook 5 minutes, stirring to brown each side. Add remaining ingredients and stir to combine.
3. Reduce heat to medium-low and simmer 1½ hours or until chicken is cooked through and tender. Remove from heat and allow to cool 1 hour.
4. Divide evenly into six airtight containers. Store in refrigerator up to 1 week, or in freezer up to 3 months, until ready to eat.
5. To serve, transfer to a saucepan and cook over medium heat 5 minutes, or microwave 1 minute, or until heated through.

THIGHS VERSUS BREASTS

Because chicken thighs are dark meat, they're juicier than chicken breasts and have a richer flavor. While most of the nutrition facts are the same, they do have a different fat content. A 4-ounce chicken thigh has 10 grams of fat, of which 2.5 grams is saturated. The same size chicken breast has 4 grams of fat, of which 1.1 grams is saturated. If you need to lower the fat macros of any chicken recipes, using chicken breasts instead of chicken thighs will make a considerable difference.

African Peanut Stew

SERVES 6

Per Serving:

Calories	621
Fat	35g
Sodium	721mg
Carbohydrates	23g
Fiber	7g
Sugar	7g
Protein	54g

Bone-in chicken thighs not only help this stew develop a richer flavor as it cooks, but they're often also one of the cheapest cuts of meat (at least as far as chicken goes). If you happen to run into some packs on sale, scoop them up and freeze them to make additional batches of this soup down the road.

2 tablespoons extra-virgin olive oil, divided

2½ pounds bone-in, skin-on chicken thighs

1 large yellow onion, peeled and diced

1 tablespoon minced fresh ginger

6 cloves garlic, peeled and minced

1 large sweet potato, peeled and cubed

1 (15-ounce) can diced tomatoes, including juice

2 tablespoons tomato paste

4 cups chicken broth

¾ cup no-sugar-added creamy peanut butter

½ cup crushed peanuts

1 teaspoon ground coriander

1 teaspoon sea salt

½ teaspoon ground black pepper

½ teaspoon ground cumin

½ teaspoon cayenne pepper

3 cups chopped collard greens

1. Heat 1 tablespoon oil in a large stockpot or Dutch oven over medium-high heat. Add chicken and cook 2 minutes on each side to brown. Remove from pot and transfer to plate.
2. Add remaining 1 tablespoon oil to pot. Add onion, ginger, and garlic and cook 4 minutes or until onion turns translucent.
3. Add remaining ingredients, except collard greens, and stir. Reduce heat to low and simmer 1½ hours or until chicken is cooked and sweet potatoes are tender.
4. Scoop chicken out of pot with a slotted spoon and set aside on a large plate to cool 5 minutes. Remove skin and bones, shred meat with two forks, and return meat to pot. Stir in collard greens. Stir, then remove from heat and allow to cool 1 hour.
5. Divide evenly into six airtight containers. Store in refrigerator up to 1 week, or in freezer up to 3 months, until ready to eat.
6. To serve, transfer to a saucepan and cook over medium heat 5 minutes, or microwave 1 minute, or until heated through.

Smoky Lentil Stew

If you want to shave some fat off this recipe, you can omit the bacon and use a little bit of avocado oil cooking spray to coat the pan before cooking the onion, carrots, and celery. The bacon does give this stew a nice smoky flavor, though, so if you can swing it, it's worth it!

SERVES 6

Per Serving:

Calories	160
Fat	2g
Sodium	517mg
Carbohydrates	23g
Fiber	8g
Sugar	6g
Protein	13g

3 slices no-sugar-added bacon, chopped

1 small yellow onion, peeled and diced

2 large carrots, peeled and diced

1 medium stalk celery, diced

3 cloves garlic, peeled and minced

2 tablespoons tomato paste

2 tablespoons smoked paprika

½ teaspoon ground cumin

1¼ cups dried red lentils, rinsed

4 cups chicken broth

1 teaspoon sea salt

½ teaspoon ground black pepper

1 tablespoon lemon juice

1. Cook bacon in a large stockpot or Dutch oven over medium-high heat until crispy, about 7 minutes. Add onion, carrots, and celery and cook until carrots start to soften, about 5 minutes. Add garlic and cook another 2 minutes. Stir in tomato paste.
2. Sprinkle paprika and cumin on top of vegetables and stir well. Cook 2 minutes. Add lentils, broth, salt, and pepper and reduce heat to medium-low. Simmer 25 minutes or until lentils reach desired level of doneness. Remove from heat and stir in lemon juice. Allow to cool 1 hour.
3. Divide evenly into six airtight containers. Store in refrigerator up to 1 week, or in freezer up to 3 months, until ready to eat.
4. To serve, transfer to a saucepan and cook over medium heat 5 minutes, or microwave 1 minute, or until heated through.

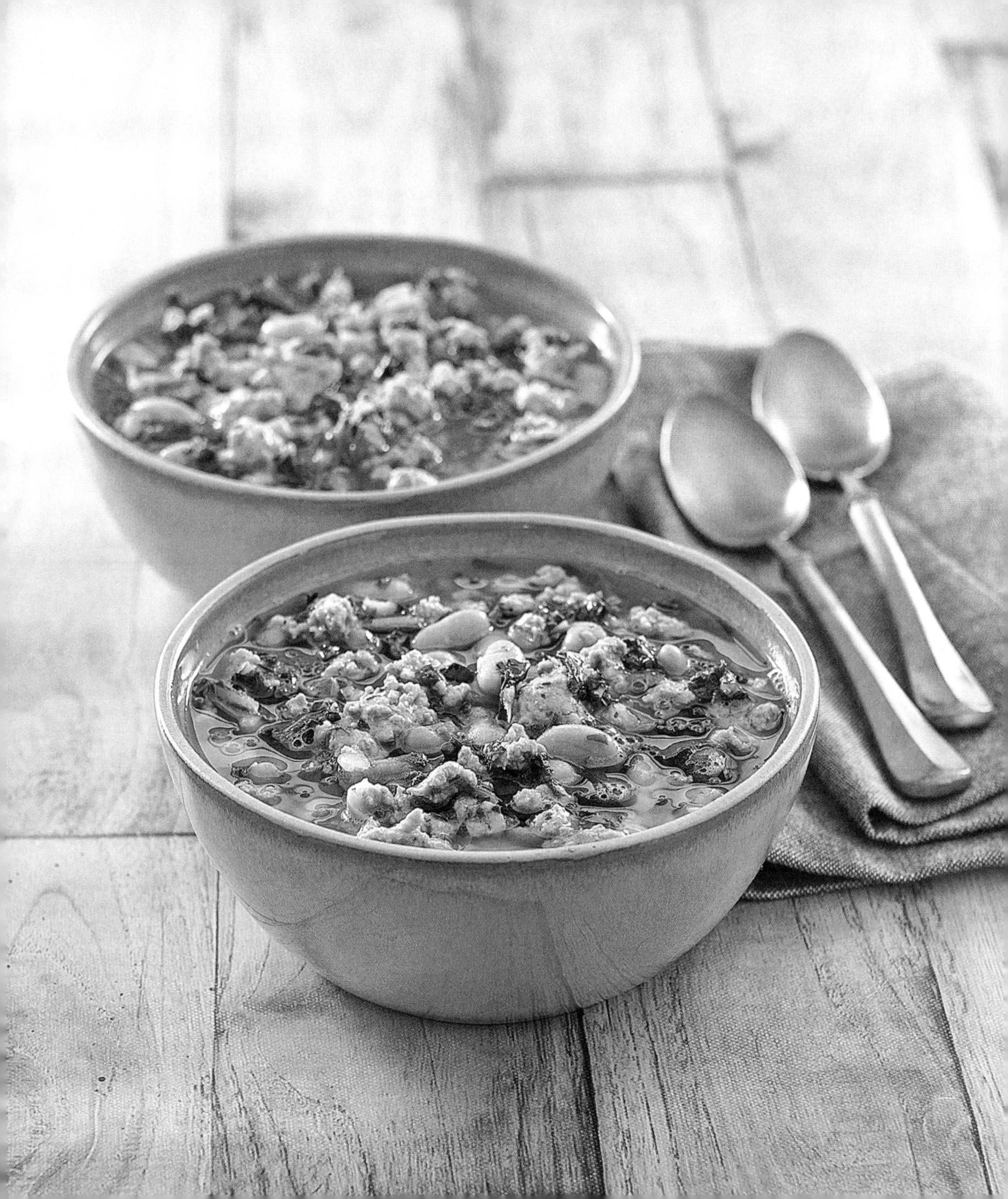

White Bean, Kale, and Sausage Soup

If you want to save on carbs, you can omit the beans without negatively affecting the recipe. To increase the protein content, add extra pork instead of the beans. To up the fiber content, double up on the kale.

SERVES 6

Per Serving:

Calories	488
Fat	34g
Sodium	531mg
Carbohydrates	17g
Fiber	5g
Sugar	2g
Protein	28g

- **2 teaspoons salt, divided**
- **1¼ teaspoons ground black pepper, divided**
- **¾ teaspoon red pepper flakes, divided**
- **½ teaspoon dried parsley**
- **¼ teaspoon ground sage**
- **¼ teaspoon dried thyme**
- **¼ teaspoon ground coriander**
- **⅛ teaspoon cayenne pepper**
- **1½ pounds ground pork**
- **1 tablespoon extra-virgin olive oil**
- **1 large yellow onion, peeled and diced**
- **2 tablespoons minced garlic**
- **4 cups chicken broth**
- **½ cup dry white wine**
- **¼ cup chopped fresh parsley**
- **3 cups frozen chopped kale**
- **1 (15-ounce) can cannellini beans, drained and rinsed**

1. Combine 1 teaspoon salt, ¼ teaspoon black pepper, ¼ teaspoon red pepper flakes, and remaining spices and herbs in a large bowl. Add pork and thoroughly mix.
2. Set pressure cooker to Sauté function and heat up oil. Add pork and cook until starting to brown, about 5 minutes. Add onion and garlic and cook until softened, about 3 minutes.
3. Stir in remaining ingredients, including remaining 1 teaspoon salt, 1 teaspoon black pepper, and ½ teaspoon red pepper flakes. Close pressure cooker lid, switch to Soup setting, and set time for 20 minutes. When time is up, allow pressure to release naturally. Open lid and allow soup to cool 1 hour.
4. Divide evenly into six airtight containers. Store in refrigerator up to 1 week, or in freezer up to 3 months, until ready to eat.
5. To serve, transfer to a saucepan and cook over medium heat 5 minutes, or microwave 1 minute, or until heated through.

FRESH TO DRIED

You can use dried herbs in place of fresh herbs in any recipe that calls for them. You do have to change the amount though, since dried herbs are more potent and concentrated. For every 1 tablespoon of fresh herbs called for in a recipe, use 1 teaspoon of dried herbs.

White Chicken Chili

SERVES 6

Per Serving:

Calories	327
Fat	7g
Sodium	688mg
Carbohydrates	28g
Fiber	11g
Sugar	3g
Protein	34g

If you have some carbs to spare, you can stir in a can of corn kernels to add a little sweetness to this chili. If you have extra fat macros instead, stir in a bit of cream cheese after cooking to thicken it up and add some extra creaminess.

1 pound boneless, skinless chicken breasts

2 teaspoons ground cumin

1 teaspoon sea salt

½ teaspoon ground black pepper

4 cups no-sugar-added chicken broth

2 (15-ounce) cans cannellini beans, drained and rinsed

1 (15-ounce) can green enchilada sauce

¾ cup shredded pepper Jack cheese

1. Put chicken in slow cooker. Sprinkle with cumin, salt, and pepper. Pour in broth, beans, and enchilada sauce. Stir to combine.
2. Cover and cook on low 6 hours or until chicken shreds easily with a fork. Remove chicken from slow cooker and transfer to a plate. Shred meat with two forks. Return meat to slow cooker and stir to combine. Cover and cook 30 minutes. Turn off slow cooker and allow to cool 1 hour.
3. Divide evenly into six airtight containers. Cover and store in refrigerator up to 1 week, or in freezer up to 3 months, until ready to eat.
4. When ready to serve, heat in a saucepan over medium-low heat 5 minutes or until heated through, then top with 2 tablespoons cheese.

Thai Coconut Curry Butternut Squash Soup

To make your meal prep even easier, you can purchase precut butternut squash at the store. (You'd need about 3 cups.) It costs a bit more than the unprepared squash, but if you can work it into your budget, it may be worth the time saved, especially if you're prepping a lot of meals in one day.

SERVES 6

Per Serving:

Calories	152
Fat	8g
Sodium	217mg
Carbohydrates	15g
Fiber	3g
Sugar	3g
Protein	4g

1 tablespoon avocado oil

1 small sweet onion, peeled and finely diced

1 large butternut squash, peeled, seeded, and cut into 1" cubes

1 tablespoon curry powder

½ teaspoon sea salt

½ teaspoon ground cinnamon

1 (14-ounce) can light coconut milk

3 cups chicken broth

1. Heat oil over medium heat in a large stockpot or Dutch oven. Add onion and cook 2 minutes. Add squash and cook another 5 minutes.
2. Stir in remaining ingredients and bring to a boil. Reduce heat to low and simmer 45 minutes. Remove from heat and use an immersion blender to purée until creamy. Allow to cool 1 hour.
3. Divide evenly into six airtight containers. Store in refrigerator up to 1 week, or in freezer up to 3 months, until ready to eat.
4. To serve, transfer to a saucepan and cook over medium heat 5 minutes, or microwave 1 minute, or until heated through.

CHAPTER 5

Poultry Main Meals

Salsa Chicken

SERVES 6

Per Serving:

Calories	189
Fat	5g
Sodium	604mg
Carbohydrates	8g
Fiber	0g
Sugar	2g
Protein	28g

BE DILIGENT ABOUT LABEL READING

When you're following a macro diet, you should be diligent about checking labels and reading ingredient lists. Added sugar lurks in places you'd least expect it, like salsa, ketchup, broth, bacon, and many other jarred and packaged foods. If a specific item contains less than 0.5 grams of sugar per serving, the food manufacturer is allowed to list it as 0 grams on the nutrition facts label, so make sure you're looking at the ingredient list. While 0.5 grams may not seem like a lot, it can add up if you're consuming more than one serving.

If you have some fat macros to spare, you can top your Salsa Chicken with a scoop of sour cream and some black olives. You can also use Greek yogurt in place of sour cream to get added creaminess and more protein.

1½ tablespoons chili powder
2 teaspoons ground cumin
1½ teaspoons sea salt
1½ teaspoons ground black pepper
1 teaspoon paprika
½ teaspoon dried oregano
½ teaspoon red pepper flakes
½ teaspoon garlic powder
½ teaspoon onion powder
6 (4-ounce) boneless, skinless chicken breasts
1½ cups no-sugar-added salsa
¾ cup shredded Cheddar cheese

1. Preheat oven to 350°F.
2. Add spices to a gallon-sized zip-top bag and shake to mix. Add chicken to bag and shake to completely coat each breast with spice mixture.
3. Put chicken in a single layer in a 9" × 13" baking dish. Top each breast with ¼ cup salsa.
4. Bake 25 minutes, add 2 tablespoons cheese to each breast, and cook another 5 minutes or until cheese is melted. Remove from oven and allow to cool 30 minutes.
5. Transfer each breast to an airtight container and store in refrigerator until ready to eat, up to 1 week.
6. To serve, transfer to a baking dish and bake at 300°F 15 minutes or until heated through.

Garlic Chicken Meatballs with Cauliflower Rice

Meatballs are an excellent choice for meal prep because you can make double or triple batches in advance and keep them in the freezer to eat later.

SERVES 6

Per Serving (4 meatballs):

Calories	196
Fat	9g
Sodium	788mg
Carbohydrates	3g
Fiber	0g
Sugar	0g
Protein	26g

FOR MEATBALLS

- 1 tablespoon extra-virgin olive oil
- 1 small yellow onion, peeled and minced
- 6 cloves garlic, peeled and minced
- 1½ pounds 98% lean ground chicken
- 1 large egg, lightly beaten
- 1 teaspoon sea salt
- ½ teaspoon ground black pepper
- 1 tablespoon grated Parmesan cheese
- 1 tablespoon Worcestershire sauce

FOR CAULIFLOWER RICE

- ¼ cup chicken broth
- 2 (12-ounce) bags cauliflower rice
- 1 teaspoon garlic powder
- 1 teaspoon sea salt
- ½ teaspoon ground black pepper
- ¼ cup chopped fresh parsley

1. To make Meatballs: Preheat oven to 400°F. Line a baking sheet with parchment paper.
2. Heat oil in a medium skillet over medium-high heat. Add onion and cook 3 minutes. Add garlic and cook another 2 minutes.
3. Transfer to a large mixing bowl. Add chicken, egg, salt, pepper, Parmesan, and Worcestershire and use your hands to mix well. Form mixture into twenty-four balls and arrange on prepared baking sheet. Bake 20 minutes or until meatballs are cooked through.
4. To make Cauliflower Rice: Combine broth and cauliflower rice in a medium saucepan over medium-high heat. Cover and cook 5 minutes or until cauliflower starts to soften. Add garlic powder, salt, and pepper and cook another 5 minutes. Stir in parsley and cook 2 more minutes or until excess liquid is absorbed.
5. Scoop equal portions of Cauliflower Rice into each of six airtight containers. Add four Meatballs to each container. Cover and store in refrigerator until ready to eat, up to 1 week.
6. To serve, transfer to a skillet and cook over medium-low heat 5 minutes or until heated through.

Lemon Pepper Chicken with Roasted Vegetables

SERVES 6

Per Serving:

Calories	170
Fat	3g
Sodium	352mg
Carbohydrates	11g
Fiber	2g
Sugar	6g
Protein	25g

This is a simple one-sheet dish that's easy to double for quick meal prep. If zucchini and summer squash aren't in season, you can switch it up by using whatever vegetables you have on-hand—just make sure to recalculate the macros accordingly.

1½ pounds boneless, skinless chicken breasts, cut into 1" cubes
2 large zucchini, cut into quarter moons
1 large summer squash, cut into quarter moons
1 medium yellow bell pepper, seeded and chopped
1 cup halved grape tomatoes
½ cup Noble Made Citrus Herb Marinade and Cooking Sauce
2 teaspoons lemon pepper

1. Preheat oven to 450°F. Line a baking sheet with parchment paper.
2. Arrange chicken, zucchini, squash, bell pepper, and tomatoes on prepared baking sheet. Drizzle with marinade, then toss to coat. Spread out in an even layer. Sprinkle lemon pepper on top.
3. Bake 25 minutes or until chicken is no longer pink and vegetables are tender. Remove from oven and allow to cool 30 minutes.
4. Divide evenly into six airtight containers. Cover and store in refrigerator until ready to eat, up to 1 week.
5. To serve, transfer to a skillet and cook over medium-low heat 5 minutes or until heated through.

Curried Chicken Thighs

If you want to cut back on fat, you can use boneless, skinless chicken breasts instead of chicken thighs. You can also drop down to nonfat Greek yogurt.

SERVES 6

Per Serving:

Calories	226
Fat	10g
Sodium	502mg
Carbohydrates	5g
Fiber	1g
Sugar	2g
Protein	29g

2 small red onions, peeled and roughly chopped
6 cloves garlic, peeled
1" knob ginger, peeled
2 tablespoons tomato paste
1 tablespoon Swerve brown sweetener
2 teaspoons garam masala
1 teaspoon sea salt
1 teaspoon ground cumin
1 teaspoon turmeric
½ teaspoon paprika
¼ teaspoon cayenne pepper
¼ cup chicken broth
1½ pounds boneless, skinless chicken thighs, cut into 1" cubes
¼ cup 2% plain Greek yogurt

1. Add onion, garlic, ginger, tomato paste, sweetener, garam masala, salt, cumin, turmeric, paprika, cayenne pepper, and broth to a food processor and process until smooth, about 40 seconds.
2. Transfer mixture to a slow cooker and stir in chicken. Cover and cook on low 5 hours. Turn off slow cooker and stir in yogurt.
3. Divide evenly into six airtight containers. Cover and store in refrigerator up to 1 week, or in freezer up to 3 months, until ready to eat.
4. To serve, transfer to a baking dish and bake at 300°F 15 minutes or until heated through.

GREEK YOGURT VERSUS REGULAR YOGURT

Greek yogurt is made by straining regular yogurt, which removes the liquid whey and some of the lactose, or milk sugar. The result is not only thicker and creamier than regular yogurt; it's higher in protein too. A cup of Greek yogurt contains about 25 grams of protein, while a cup of regular yogurt has 14 grams.

Garlic Sesame Chicken Thighs

SERVES 6

Per Serving:

Calories	217
Fat	9g
Sodium	285mg
Carbohydrates	10g
Fiber	0g
Sugar	1g
Protein	25g

A WORD ON SWERVE

Swerve is a low-carb, keto-friendly sweetener that's made with erythritol (a sugar alcohol) and prebiotic fibers called oligosaccharides. While the nutrition facts label says that Swerve contains 4 grams of carbohydrates per teaspoon, all 4 grams of these carbohydrates come from the sugar alcohols and fiber. That means that they have no effect on your blood sugar levels and technically don't count toward your macros.

If you want to drop the fat in this recipe a little bit, you can use chicken breasts in place of chicken thighs. Make it as is if you can spare the extra fat grams, though. The thighs add a lot of flavor and make this dish feel really authentic.

2 pounds boneless, skinless chicken thighs
½ cup coconut aminos
4 cloves garlic, peeled and minced
1 tablespoon grated fresh ginger
¼ cup Tessemae's Unsweetened Ketchup
2 teaspoons sriracha
¼ cup Swerve brown sweetener
1 tablespoon toasted sesame oil
2 teaspoons arrowroot powder
2 teaspoons water
1 tablespoon sesame seeds
¼ cup chopped scallions

1. Add chicken, coconut aminos, garlic, ginger, ketchup, and sriracha to pressure cooker and stir to combine. Close the lid, set to manual/high pressure, and set time for 3 minutes. When time is up, manually release pressure.
2. Carefully open lid. Set pressure cooker to Sauté and add sweetener and oil. Stir to combine.
3. Whisk arrowroot and water in a small bowl until smooth. Stir mixture into pressure cooker and continue cooking, stirring continuously, 5 minutes or until sauce thickens. Turn off pressure cooker. Allow to cool 30 minutes.
4. Divide evenly into six airtight containers. Sprinkle sesame seeds and scallions on top. Cover and store in refrigerator until ready to eat, up to 1 week.
5. To serve, transfer to a skillet and cook over medium-low heat 5 minutes or until heated through.

Ground Turkey Cabbage Roll Casserole

It's best to use freshly grated cauliflower rice, but if you use frozen, let it defrost first and then squeeze out any excess liquid before proceeding with the rest of this recipe. It will still work if you use the frozen cauliflower rice without defrosting, but it will be a little soggy.

SERVES 6

Per Serving:

Calories	433
Fat	27g
Sodium	1,008mg
Carbohydrates	18g
Fiber	5g
Sugar	8g
Protein	33g

- 1 tablespoon avocado oil
- 3 cloves garlic, peeled and minced
- 2 small shallots, peeled and minced
- 1½ pounds 90% lean ground turkey
- 1 teaspoon sea salt
- ½ teaspoon ground black pepper
- 4 cups cauliflower rice
- 6 cups shredded cabbage
- 1½ tablespoons Italian seasoning
- 1 teaspoon dried basil
- 1 teaspoon dried parsley
- ¼ teaspoon red pepper flakes
- 3½ cups no-sugar-added pizza sauce
- 2 cups shredded mozzarella cheese

1. Preheat oven to 350°F.
2. Heat oil in a large stockpot or Dutch oven over medium-high heat. Add garlic and shallots and cook 3 minutes. Add turkey, salt, and pepper and cook until no longer pink, about 10 minutes.
3. While turkey is cooking, mix cauliflower and cabbage together in a medium bowl. Sprinkle Italian seasoning, basil, parsley, and red pepper flakes on top and toss to coat evenly.
4. Add cabbage mixture to turkey mixture and stir to mix. Pour in pizza sauce and stir until incorporated. Cook 2 minutes.
5. Transfer mixture to a 9" × 13" baking dish. Sprinkle cheese on top.
6. Cover with aluminum foil and bake 10 minutes or until cabbage starts to soften. Remove foil and bake another 15 minutes until casserole is bubbly and cheese starts to turn golden brown. Remove from oven and allow to cool 1 hour.
7. Divide evenly into six airtight containers. Cover and store in refrigerator up to 1 week, or in freezer up to 3 months, until ready to eat.
8. To serve, transfer to a skillet and cook over medium-low heat 5 minutes or until heated through.

IS GROUND TURKEY A SUITABLE REPLACEMENT FOR GROUND BEEF?

Ground turkey is one of the leanest (meaning lowest in fat) ground meats that you can buy. It's a suitable replacement for ground beef in any recipe, but since it does have less fat, it's not as juicy. Because of this, you'll have to watch cooking times closely and make sure you're not overcooking it, or it will be dry and chewy. If you use ground turkey in place of beef in a recipe, you may also need to throw in some additional spices since you'll lose some of the flavor that comes from the fat in beef.

Caprese Chicken with Roasted Tomatoes

SERVES 6

Per Serving:

Calories	254
Fat	10g
Sodium	635mg
Carbohydrates	8g
Fiber	1g
Sugar	4g
Protein	32g

Rather than buying sliced mozzarella cheese from the deli, grab a fresh mozzarella ball and use that instead. It makes a big difference in the outcome of this dish.

FOR TOMATOES

- 1 pound cherry tomatoes, halved
- 2 teaspoons extra-virgin olive oil
- 3 cloves garlic, peeled and minced
- ½ teaspoon sea salt
- ¼ teaspoon ground black pepper
- ¼ teaspoon red pepper flakes

FOR CHICKEN

- 6 (4-ounce) boneless, skinless chicken breasts
- 1 tablespoon extra-virgin olive oil
- 1 teaspoon granulated garlic
- 1 teaspoon Italian seasoning
- 1 teaspoon sea salt
- ½ teaspoon ground black pepper
- 12 slices large beefsteak tomato
- 6 slices fresh mozzarella (from an 8-ounce mozzarella ball)
- 6 tablespoons balsamic vinegar
- 12 fresh basil leaves

1. To make Tomatoes: Preheat oven to 350°F. Spray a 9" × 13" baking dish with avocado oil cooking spray.
2. Put cherry tomatoes in a large bowl. Add remaining ingredients and toss to coat. Spread out in prepared baking dish.
3. To make Chicken: Arrange chicken in a single layer on top of Tomatoes. Drizzle with oil and sprinkle with garlic, Italian seasoning, salt, and pepper. Layer 2 beefsteak tomato slices on top of each breast.
4. Bake 25 minutes or until chicken reaches an internal temperature of 165°F. Place 1 mozzarella slice on top of each breast and bake 1 more minute. Remove from oven and allow to cool 30 minutes.
5. Transfer Chicken to each of six airtight containers. Add a scoop of roasted Tomatoes to each container. Drizzle 1 tablespoon vinegar on top of each breast and top with 2 basil leaves.
6. Cover and store in refrigerator until ready to eat, up to 1 week.
7. To serve, transfer to a skillet and cook over medium-low heat 5 minutes or until heated through.

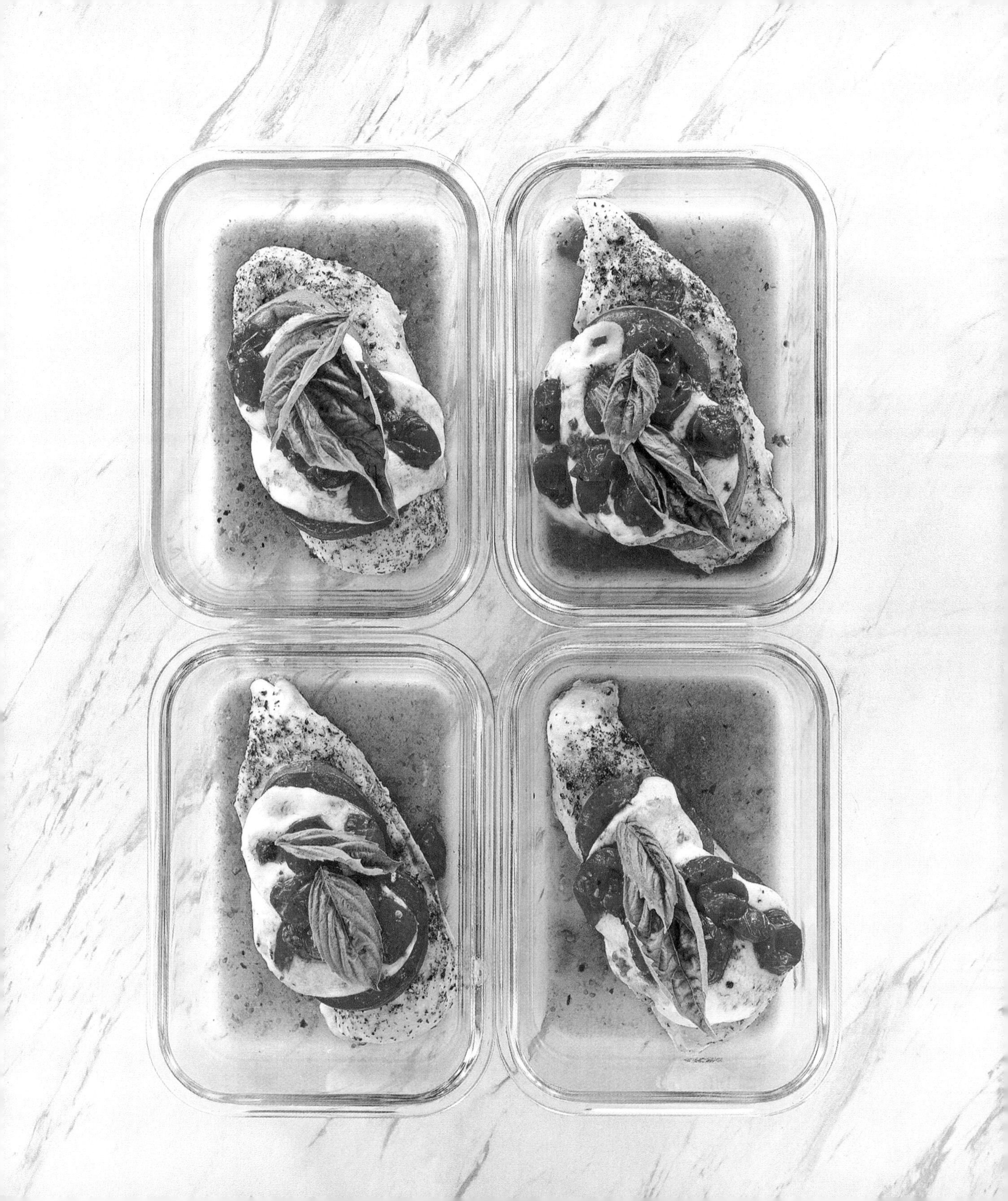

One-Pan Pesto Chicken with Vegetables

SERVES 6

Per Serving:

Calories	192
Fat	8g
Sodium	738mg
Carbohydrates	5g
Fiber	1g
Sugar	2g
Protein	24g

This recipe is an excellent way to use up any extra vegetables that you have in your refrigerator at the end of the week. Feel free to get creative and play around with different combinations.

1 tablespoon extra-virgin olive oil
1½ pounds chicken tenders
½ cup chopped sun-dried tomatoes
2 cloves garlic, peeled and minced
½ teaspoon sea salt
2 cups chopped Swiss chard
⅓ cup basil pesto
1 cup halved cherry tomatoes

1. Heat oil in a large skillet over medium heat. Add chicken, sun-dried tomatoes, garlic, and salt and cook 8 minutes, flipping once during cooking, until chicken is no longer pink.
2. Stir in Swiss chard, cover, and cook until wilted, about 2 minutes. Stir in pesto and cherry tomatoes and cook 1 more minute. Remove from heat and allow to cool 30 minutes.
3. Transfer equal parts of chicken and vegetable mixture to each of six airtight containers. Store in refrigerator until ready to eat, up to 1 week.
4. To serve, transfer to a skillet and cook over medium-low heat 5 minutes or until heated through.

Buffalo Chicken–Stuffed Peppers

You can use any color bell peppers you want for these stuffed peppers, but the natural sweetness of the orange bell peppers goes really well with the spiciness of the buffalo sauce in this recipe.

SERVES 6

Per Serving:

Calories	170
Fat	2g
Sodium	248mg
Carbohydrates	11g
Fiber	2g
Sugar	5g
Protein	27g

6 (4-ounce) boneless, skinless chicken breasts
1 medium yellow onion, peeled and sliced
1 teaspoon dried parsley
1 teaspoon dried dill
1 teaspoon dried chives
1 teaspoon garlic powder
1 teaspoon onion powder
½ teaspoon sea salt
½ teaspoon ground black pepper
¾ cup Noble Made Medium Buffalo Sauce
6 medium orange bell peppers, tops cut off, seeded

1. Preheat oven to 350°F. Line a baking sheet with parchment paper.
2. Arrange chicken and sliced onion in a single layer on prepared baking sheet. Sprinkle evenly with spices. Bake 30 minutes or until chicken is no longer pink.
3. Remove from oven and cut chicken and onion into bite-sized pieces. Transfer to a large bowl and combine with buffalo sauce. Scoop equal parts chicken mixture evenly into each bell pepper.
4. Stand bell peppers up in a 9" × 9" baking dish and bake 30 minutes or until peppers are softened. Remove from oven and allow to cool 30 minutes.
5. Transfer each pepper to an airtight container and store in refrigerator until ready to eat, up to 1 week.
6. To serve, transfer to a baking dish and bake at 300°F 20 minutes or until heated through.

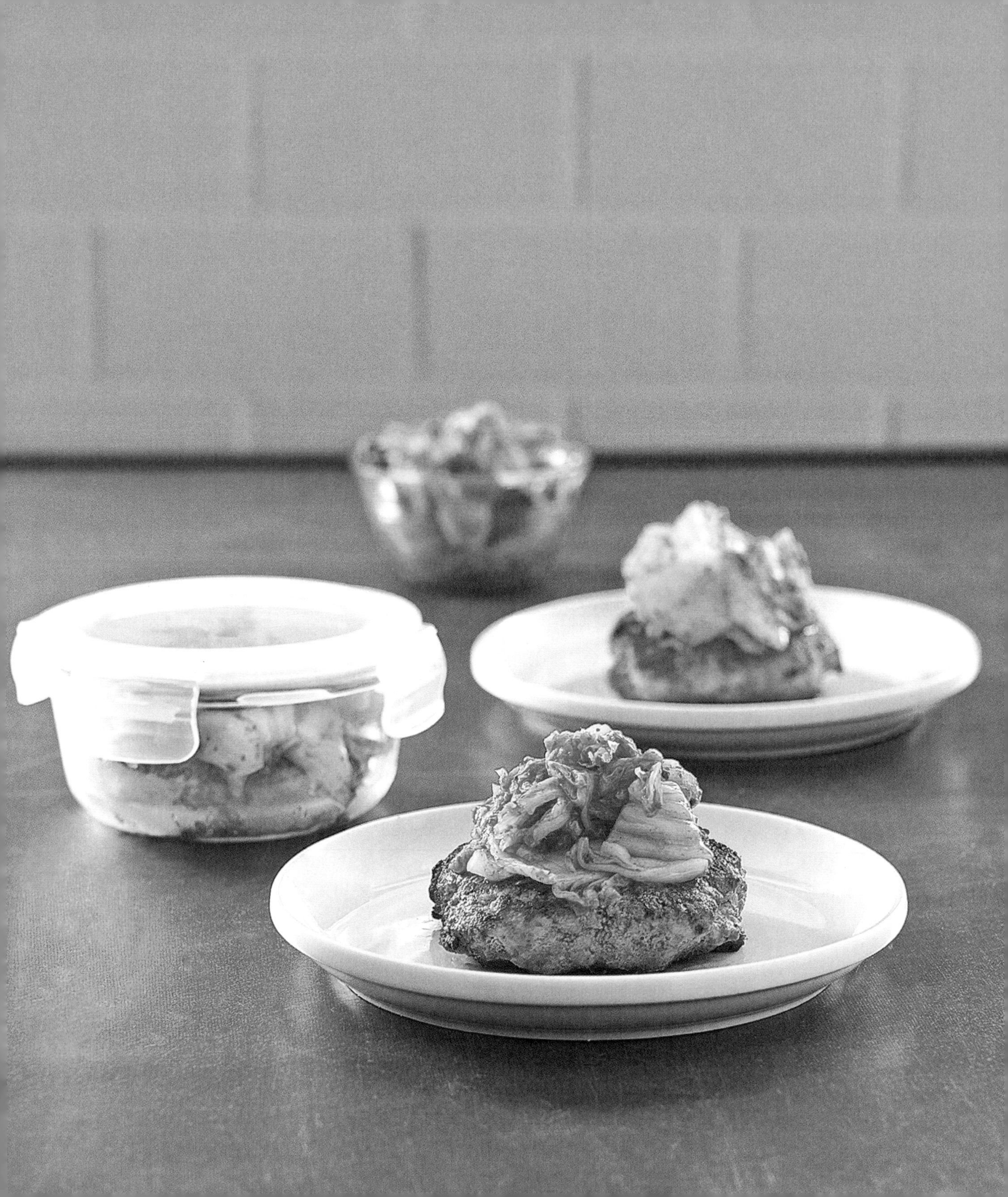

Turkey Burgers with Kimchi

Kimchi not only adds a delightful tangy, spicy flavor to this dish; it's also loaded with probiotics that help keep your gut healthy and functioning properly. If you can't find kimchi, you can use a high-quality sauerkraut for a similar taste and health benefit.

SERVES 6

Per Serving:

Calories	216
Fat	14g
Sodium	721mg
Carbohydrates	3g
Fiber	0g
Sugar	1g
Protein	19g

1½ pounds 90% lean ground turkey

1 teaspoon sea salt

½ teaspoon ground black pepper

1 tablespoon Tessemae's Unsweetened Ketchup

2 teaspoons Worcestershire sauce

2 cloves garlic, peeled and minced

1 tablespoon extra-virgin olive oil

¾ cup Wildbrine Korean Kimchi

1. Combine turkey, salt, pepper, ketchup, Worcestershire, and garlic in a large bowl. Form into six equal patties.
2. Heat oil in a large skillet over medium heat. Add turkey patties and cook 4 minutes on each side or until no longer pink. Remove from heat and allow to cool 30 minutes.
3. Transfer burgers to each of six airtight containers. Top each burger with 2 tablespoons kimchi. Cover and store in refrigerator until ready to eat, up to 1 week.
4. To serve, transfer to a skillet and cook, covered, over medium-low heat 5 minutes or until heated through. Or serve cold.

Spinach and Feta Chicken Patties

SERVES 6

Per Serving:

Calories	236
Fat	14g
Sodium	497mg
Carbohydrates	2g
Fiber	1g
Sugar	1g
Protein	27g

Make sure the frozen spinach is squeezed dry before mixing it with the other ingredients in this recipe. It will prevent the chicken patties from getting soggy and keep them from falling apart. Use a cheesecloth or a nut bag to get all the excess liquid out.

1½ pounds 93% lean ground turkey

2 large eggs, lightly beaten

1½ teaspoons minced garlic

⅓ cup crumbled feta cheese

1 (10-ounce) package frozen chopped spinach, thawed and squeezed dry

¾ teaspoon sea salt

½ teaspoon ground black pepper

2 teaspoons coconut aminos

2 tablespoons avocado oil

1. Combine all ingredients, except oil, in a large bowl and mix until just incorporated. Form mixture into six equal patties.
2. Heat oil in a large skillet over medium-high heat. Cook patties 4 minutes, flip, and cook for an additional 4 minutes or until chicken is no longer pink. Remove from heat and allow to cool 30 minutes.
3. Transfer each patty to an airtight container and store in refrigerator until ready to eat, up to 1 week.
4. To serve, transfer to a skillet and cook over medium-low heat 5 minutes, flipping once during cooking, or until heated through.

Firecracker Chicken

This spicy dish is made with ground chicken and comes together in minutes. While it's easy enough to whip up for a week's worth of meals, you can also double up the batch and freeze some for later for easy meal prep.

SERVES 6

Per Serving:

Calories	199
Fat	5g
Sodium	651mg
Carbohydrates	17g
Fiber	0g
Sugar	0g
Protein	22g

½ cup Swerve brown sweetener
¼ cup Noble Made Medium Buffalo Sauce
2 tablespoons unsweetened applesauce
2 tablespoons apple cider vinegar
1 teaspoon sea salt
½ teaspoon ground black pepper
1 teaspoon garlic powder
½ teaspoon ground ginger
½ teaspoon red pepper flakes
1 teaspoon avocado oil
1½ pounds 93% lean ground chicken

1. Add sweetener, buffalo sauce, applesauce, vinegar, salt, black pepper, garlic powder, ginger, and red pepper flakes to a medium bowl and whisk until smooth. Set aside.
2. Heat oil in a large skillet over medium heat. Add chicken and cook until no longer pink, about 8 minutes. Pour sauce over chicken and stir to coat. Cook 1 more minute. Remove from heat.
3. Divide evenly into six airtight containers. Cover and store in refrigerator up to 1 week, or in freezer up to 3 months, until ready to eat.
4. To serve, transfer to a skillet and cook over medium-low heat 5 minutes or until heated through.

ANOTHER WORD ON SWERVE

Thanks to its zero net carbs, and a taste that's shockingly close to regular sugar, Swerve is a convenient option for sweetening sauces or making baked goods that fit into your macros. While many people tolerate Swerve well, it does have the potential to cause some gas and bloating. If you've just started consuming Swerve and you notice your digestion seems off, cut it out or cut back on it to see if that helps normalize things. Keep in mind that it does have fiber in it, so it could just take a little while to get used to it.

Hawaiian Barbecue Chicken

SERVES 6

Per Serving:

Calories	251
Fat	8g
Sodium	962mg
Carbohydrates	30g
Fiber	1g
Sugar	11g
Protein	16g

The pineapple added to the end of this recipe gives this dish the perfect marriage of savory and sweet, but if you want to cut back on carbs you can eliminate it or reduce the amount.

¾ cup coconut aminos

¾ cup Tessemae's Unsweetened Ketchup

½ cup Swerve brown sweetener

⅓ cup chicken broth

2 teaspoons minced fresh ginger

2 teaspoons minced garlic

1½ pounds boneless, skinless chicken thighs

1 teaspoon arrowroot powder

1 teaspoon water

1 cup chopped fresh pineapple

1. Combine coconut aminos, ketchup, sweetener, broth, ginger, and garlic in a slow cooker and mix well. Add chicken and stir to coat. Cover and cook on low 5 hours.
2. Whisk arrowroot and water in a small bowl until smooth. Stir into slow cooker with pineapple. Cover and cook another 1 hour.
3. Turn off slow cooker and use two forks to shred chicken. Mix in sauce. Allow to cool 30 minutes.
4. Divide evenly into six airtight containers. Cover and store in refrigerator up to 1 week, or in freezer up to 3 months, until ready to eat.
5. To serve, transfer to a skillet and cook over medium-low heat 5 minutes or until heated through.

Turkey-Stuffed Peppers

Turkey is a lower-fat alternative to ground beef, but if you have room for beef in your macros and prefer the richer flavor, you can swap proteins. You can also mix the two and use half ground beef and half ground turkey. Just make sure to adjust the macros accordingly.

SERVES 6

Per Serving:

Calories	258
Fat	15g
Sodium	525mg
Carbohydrates	7g
Fiber	2g
Sugar	4g
Protein	22g

1 tablespoon avocado oil

1 medium yellow onion, peeled and chopped

3 cloves garlic, peeled and minced

1½ pounds 90% lean ground turkey

1 teaspoon ground cumin

1 teaspoon chili powder

1 teaspoon paprika

½ teaspoon sea salt

½ teaspoon ground black pepper

1 (14.5-ounce) can fire-roasted diced tomatoes, including juice

6 large red bell peppers, tops cut off, seeded

½ cup shredded mozzarella cheese

1. Preheat oven to 375°F.
2. Heat oil in a large skillet over medium-high heat. Add onion and garlic and sauté 3 minutes or until starting to soften.
3. Add turkey, stir in spices, and cook until turkey is no longer pink, about 6 minutes.
4. Stir in tomatoes and bring to a boil. Turn heat to low and simmer 5 minutes or until some liquid evaporates.
5. Stand bell peppers up in a 9" × 9" baking dish. Scoop equal amounts of turkey mixture into peppers. Bake 40 minutes.
6. Sprinkle cheese on top of peppers and bake another 5 minutes. Turn oven to broil and broil 2 minutes. Remove from oven and allow to cool 30 minutes.
7. Transfer stuffed peppers to each of six airtight containers and store in refrigerator until ready to eat, up to 1 week.
8. To serve, transfer to a baking dish and bake at 300°F 20 minutes or until heated through.

PRECOOKING YOUR PEPPERS

When you're making stuffed peppers, it can take a while, at least 45 minutes, for the peppers to adequately soften. If you're in a rush, or just want to shorten the cooking time so you can free up your oven to prep another meal, you can precook the peppers. Simply fill up a large pot of water and submerge the peppers. Bring the water to a boil, reduce the heat, and let them simmer for about 3 minutes. Remove them from the hot water and dunk them in an ice bath. Once they're cooled off, proceed with the recipe as written.

Baked Cheddar Ranch Chicken

SERVES 6

Per Serving:

Calories	164
Fat	5g
Sodium	302mg
Carbohydrates	0g
Fiber	0g
Sugar	0g
Protein	30g

If you don't have Flavor God Ranch Topper, you might want to consider adding it to your spice cabinet (it's used in a few recipes in this book). You can replace it with another ranch seasoning, but it may change the macros slightly.

6 (4-ounce) boneless, skinless chicken breasts

2 tablespoons Flavor God Ranch Topper

½ cup shredded Cheddar cheese

1. Preheat oven to 350°F. Line a baking sheet with parchment paper.
2. Put chicken in a large zip-top bag. Add ranch seasoning and shake to coat evenly.
3. Arrange chicken in a single layer on prepared baking sheet. Bake 20 minutes. Sprinkle cheese on top and bake another 10 minutes or until cheese melts and chicken reaches an internal temperature of 165°F. Remove from oven and allow to cool 30 minutes.
4. Put a chicken breast in each of six airtight containers. Cover and store in refrigerator until ready to eat, up to 1 week.
5. To serve, transfer to a skillet and cook over medium-low heat 5 minutes or until heated through.

Buffalo Chicken Zucchini Boats

The Tessemae's Habanero Ranch dressing adds an extra kick to this recipe, but if you think the buffalo sauce makes it hot enough, you can swap it out for regular ranch or blue cheese.

SERVES 6

Per Serving (2 zucchini boats):

Calories	445
Fat	31g
Sodium	984mg
Carbohydrates	11g
Fiber	3g
Sugar	6g
Protein	31g

6 large zucchini, tops trimmed, halved lengthwise

6 tablespoons Nutiva Buttery Flavor Coconut Oil

¾ cup minced yellow onion

3 cups shredded cooked boneless, skinless chicken breasts

¾ cup Noble Made Medium Buffalo Sauce

6 tablespoons Tessemae's Habanero Ranch dressing

6 tablespoons diced avocado

1. Preheat oven to 350°F.
2. Scoop out some of the flesh in each zucchini half to create a "boat." Roughly chop scooped zucchini and set aside.
3. Heat oil in a large skillet over medium heat. Add onion and cook 2 minutes. Stir in chopped zucchini and cook another 2 minutes or until slightly softened.
4. Add chicken and stir to incorporate. Pour buffalo sauce on top of chicken mixture and stir until just combined. Remove from heat.
5. Arrange zucchini, cut-side up, in a 9" × 13" baking dish. Scoop equal amounts of buffalo chicken into each zucchini boat and spread out evenly.
6. Bake 20 minutes or until zucchini is tender. Remove from oven and allow to cool 30 minutes.
7. Transfer 2 zucchini boats to each of six airtight containers and store in refrigerator until ready to eat, up to 1 week.
8. To serve, broil zucchini boats on high 2 minutes or heat in microwave 30 seconds. Drizzle with 1 tablespoon ranch dressing and top with 1 tablespoon chopped avocado before serving.

BULK SHREDDED CHICKEN

It's helpful to make cooked chicken in bulk and freeze in batches for recipes like this. Combine 1 teaspoon salt, 1 teaspoon ground black pepper, 1 teaspoon garlic powder, and 1 teaspoon onion powder and sprinkle it over 3 pounds of boneless, skinless chicken breasts. Place chicken in slow cooker, pour 1 cup of chicken bone broth on top, cover, and cook on low for 6–8 hours. When chicken is done, shred with two forks and store in the refrigerator up to 1 week or freeze in batches.

High-Protein Chicken Alfredo

SERVES 6

Per Serving:

Calories	220
Fat	9g
Sodium	713mg
Carbohydrates	3g
Fiber	0g
Sugar	2g
Protein	32g

Thanks to the Greek yogurt, this alfredo sauce is all about the protein. If you have room for some extra carbs, you can serve this over a high-protein pasta like Banza, or you can keep it low-carb by pairing it with spaghetti squash. It's also delicious as is—no pasta needed!

FOR CHICKEN

6 (4-ounce) boneless, skinless chicken breasts

1 teaspoon garlic powder

½ teaspoon sea salt

½ teaspoon ground black pepper

FOR SAUCE

2 tablespoons unsalted grass-fed butter

2 teaspoons minced garlic

½ cup 2% organic milk

¾ cup nonfat plain Greek yogurt

½ cup shredded Parmesan cheese

1 teaspoon sea salt

½ teaspoon ground black pepper

1. To make Chicken: Preheat oven to 350°F.
2. Arrange chicken in a single layer in a 9" × 13" baking dish and sprinkle garlic powder, salt, and pepper on top. Bake 25 minutes or until chicken reaches an internal temperature of 165°F. Remove from oven and allow to cool 30 minutes.
3. To make Sauce: While chicken is cooking, melt butter in a medium saucepan over medium heat. Add garlic and cook 2 minutes. Add milk and yogurt and stir until combined. Reduce heat to low and add cheese in small batches, stirring in between, until it melts. Stir in salt and pepper. Remove from heat and allow to cool 30 minutes.
4. Transfer Chicken to each of six airtight containers. Scoop equal amounts Sauce on top. Cover and store in refrigerator up to 1 week, until ready to eat.
5. To serve, transfer to a skillet and cook over medium-low heat 5 minutes or until heated through.

Chicken Bacon Ranch Spaghetti Squash

If you need to play around with the fat in this recipe, you can reduce the amount of bacon or cut it out completely.

SERVES 4

Per Serving:

Calories	444
Fat	30g
Sodium	1,084mg
Carbohydrates	8g
Fiber	2g
Sugar	3g
Protein	33g

1 large spaghetti squash, halved lengthwise

1 pound cooked boneless, skinless chicken breasts, cut into bite-sized pieces

⅔ cup Tessemae's Creamy Ranch Dressing

¼ cup light coconut milk

2 tablespoons nutritional yeast

1 teaspoon sea salt

½ teaspoon ground black pepper

6 slices no-sugar-added bacon, cooked and crumbled

2 cups chopped fresh spinach

1 teaspoon Flavor God Ranch Topper

1. Preheat oven to 400°F. Line a baking sheet with parchment paper.
2. Put squash cut-side down on prepared baking sheet. Bake 45 minutes or until a fork slides into squash easily. Remove from oven and allow to cool 10 minutes.
3. Using a fork, shred squash and transfer to a 9" × 9" baking dish.
4. Add cooked chicken, ranch dressing, coconut milk, nutritional yeast, salt, and pepper to a medium bowl and whisk until smooth. Pour mixture over squash and stir to coat. Stir in bacon and spinach. Sprinkle ranch seasoning on top.
5. Bake 20 minutes or until sauce is hot and bubbly. Remove from oven and allow to cool 1 hour.
6. Divide evenly into six airtight containers. Cover and store in refrigerator up to 1 week, or in freezer up to 3 months, until ready to eat.
7. To serve, transfer to a skillet and cook over medium-low heat 5 minutes or until heated through.

One-Pan Chicken Piccata

SERVES 6

Per Serving:

Calories	184
Fat	9g
Sodium	441mg
Carbohydrates	0g
Fiber	0g
Sugar	0g
Protein	26g

If you want to make a full prepped meal, you can combine this chicken piccata with ½ to 1 cup cooked spaghetti squash or zucchini noodles. Just put your "noodles" in your meal prep container and then put the chicken on top and store in the refrigerator until you're ready to eat.

6 (4-ounce) boneless, skinless chicken cutlets

1 teaspoon sea salt

½ teaspoon ground black pepper

½ teaspoon garlic powder

3 tablespoons unsalted grass-fed butter

1 tablespoon extra-virgin olive oil

½ cup chicken broth

¼ cup dry white wine

3 tablespoons lemon juice

2 tablespoons capers

1. Season chicken on both sides with salt, pepper, and garlic powder.
2. Add butter and oil to a large skillet and heat over medium-high heat. Add chicken and cook 3 minutes on each side. Use tongs to transfer chicken to a plate.
3. Pour broth, wine, and lemon juice into pan and stir, scraping browned bits off bottom of pan. Bring to a boil, then reduce heat to medium.
4. Return chicken to pan and simmer 5 minutes. Remove from heat and stir in capers. Allow to cool 30 minutes.
5. Transfer chicken and sauce to each of six airtight containers. Cover and store in refrigerator until ready to eat, up to 1 week.
6. To serve, transfer to a skillet and cook over medium-low heat 5 minutes or until heated through.

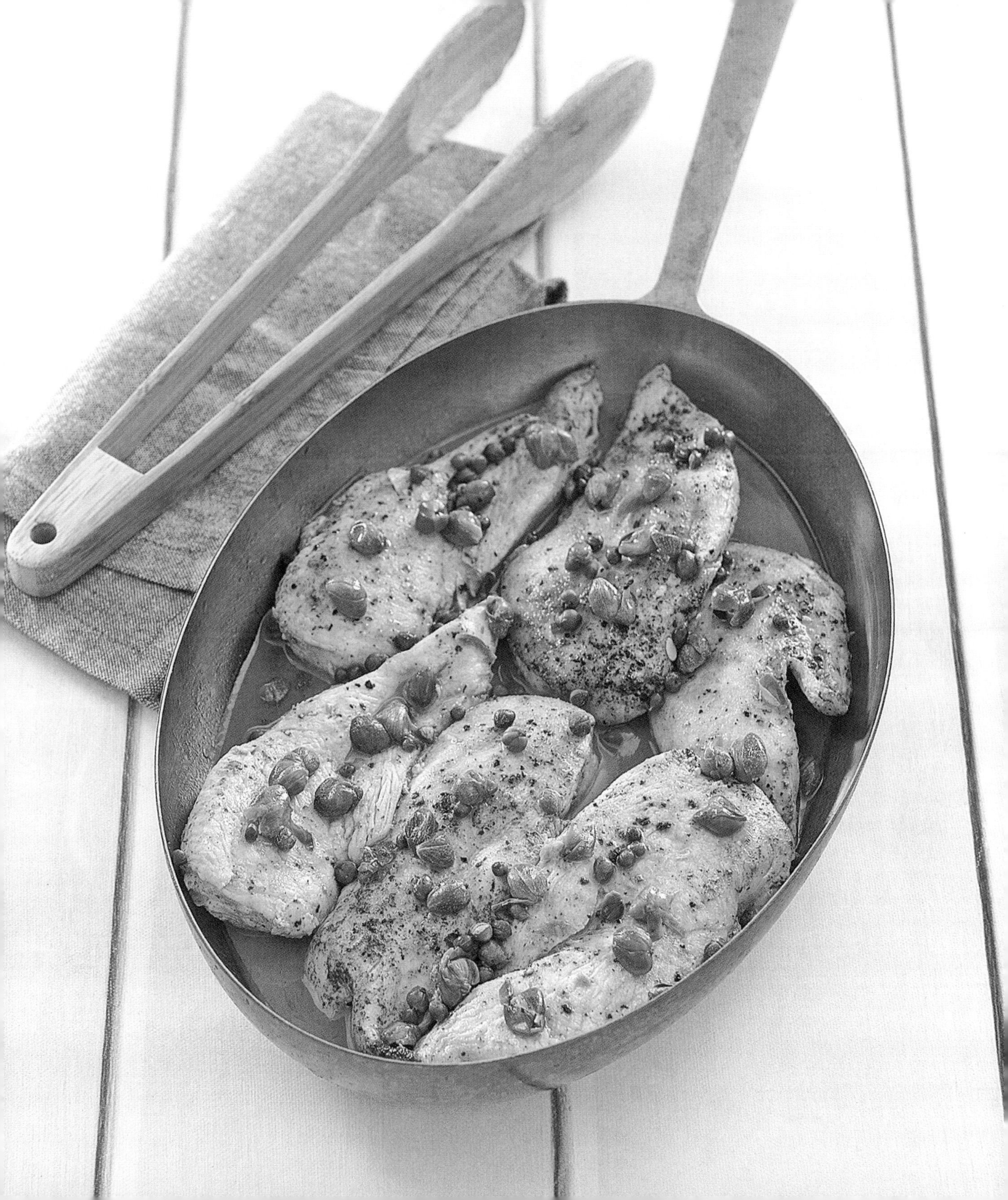

Buffalo Chicken Mac and Cheese

SERVES 6

Per Serving:

Calories	313
Fat	11g
Sodium	499mg
Carbohydrates	27g
Fiber	4g
Sugar	3g
Protein	27g

MAKE YOUR OWN CHEESE POWDER

All you need is a semisoft cheese, like Cheddar, and a dehydrator to make your own powdered cheese. Cut a cheese block into uniform slices. Arrange the slices in single layers on the dehydrator trays and dehydrate for 6 to 10 hours, until the cheese is fully dry. During the process, you might want to blot out excess fat and flip the slices once or twice. Once dry, allow cheese to fully cool, then transfer it to a food processor and pulse to a powder. Store it in an airtight container and use it to flavor anything that needs a cheese boost!

The cheese powder in this recipe really adds some depth of flavor, so try not to skip it. It's worth the extra effort to find the King Arthur brand, though, because it doesn't have a long list of artificial ingredients like other cheese powders—it's just concentrated cheese.

1 pound 93% lean ground chicken

1 small yellow onion, peeled and minced

4 cloves garlic, peeled and minced

¼ cup Noble Made Medium Buffalo Sauce

¾ cup 2% plain Greek yogurt

¼ cup King Arthur Better Cheddar Cheese Powder

8 ounces Banza pasta shells, cooked according to package instructions

1. Heat a large nonstick skillet over medium-high heat. Add chicken, onion, and garlic and cook until chicken is no longer pink, about 8 minutes. Stir in buffalo sauce and cook 3 more minutes or until mixture starts to thicken.
2. Whisk yogurt and cheese powder in a small bowl until smooth. Fold into chicken mixture and stir to mix well. Add cooked pasta and mix to coat. Allow to cool.
3. Divide evenly into six airtight containers. Cover and store in refrigerator until ready to eat, up to 1 week.
4. To serve, transfer to a skillet and cook over medium-low heat 5 minutes or until heated through.

CHAPTER 6

Beef and Pork Main Meals

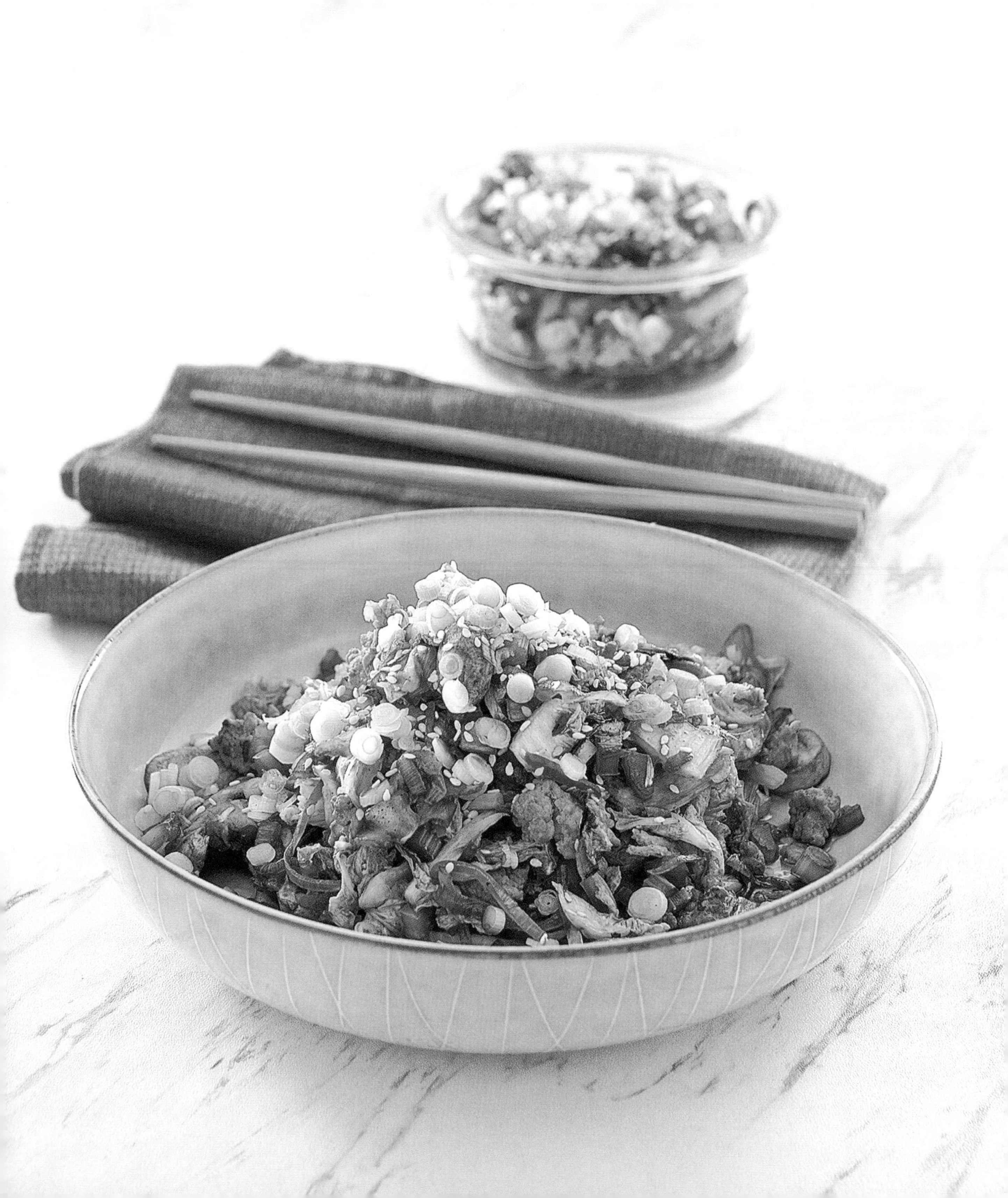

Egg Roll in a Bowl

This one-pot recipe comes together in under 20 minutes, making it an excellent choice for weeknight meal prep. If you want to cut down on the fat, you can replace the pork with ground turkey or ground chicken.

SERVES 6

Per Serving:

Calories	413
Fat	26g
Sodium	620mg
Carbohydrates	10g
Fiber	6g
Sugar	10g
Protein	23g

2 teaspoons avocado oil
1 large yellow onion, peeled and thinly sliced
1 teaspoon minced garlic
1½ pounds ground pork
4 medium stalks celery, chopped
12 cups shredded cabbage
1 cup sliced white mushrooms
⅓ cup coconut aminos
¾ teaspoon ground ginger
½ teaspoon sea salt
½ teaspoon ground black pepper
1 tablespoon beef broth
1 tablespoon sriracha
1 tablespoon toasted sesame oil
2 tablespoons chopped scallions
2 tablespoons sesame seeds

1. Heat avocado oil in a large skillet over medium-high heat. Add onion and sauté 5 minutes. Add garlic and cook 1 minute. Crumble pork into pan and cook until no longer pink, about 8 minutes.
2. Add celery, cabbage, mushrooms, coconut aminos, ginger, salt, pepper, and broth to pan and stir to combine. Cover and cook 10 minutes or until cabbage reaches desired level of tenderness. Stir in sriracha. Remove from heat and stir in sesame oil and scallions. Sprinkle sesame seeds on top.
3. Divide evenly into six airtight containers. Cover and store in refrigerator until ready to eat, up to 1 week.
4. When ready to serve, transfer to a skillet over medium heat and cook 5 minutes or until heated through.

SPEED THINGS UP WITH COLESLAW MIX

If you're short on time and don't want to shred your own cabbage, you can grab some prepackaged coleslaw mix, which is just shredded cabbage, and usually some carrots, in a bag. This route will probably cost a bit more than shredding the cabbage yourself, but it's a convenient option especially when you're prepping a lot of meals at once.

Low-Carb Patty Melts

SERVES 6

Per Serving:

Calories	376
Fat	25g
Sodium	558mg
Carbohydrates	5g
Fiber	0g
Sugar	3g
Protein	31g

THE BEST MASHED CAULIFLOWER

Mashed cauliflower is an excellent low-carb side dish that tastes just like mashed potatoes, only fluffier, if you do it right. Boil cauliflower florets for 10 minutes or until tender. Drain cauliflower and transfer to a food processor with 2 tablespoons unsalted butter, 1 teaspoon garlic powder, ¾ teaspoon sea salt, and ½ teaspoon ground black pepper and process until smooth. Taste and adjust spices accordingly. Enjoy with your patty melt.

These patty melts are made bun-free to keep the carb count low. If you have some carbs to spare, you can pop them on your favorite macro-friendly bun after reheating. Otherwise, if you want to keep the meal low-carb, serve them on top of a bed of greens or with mashed cauliflower on the side.

FOR PATTY MELTS

- 2 teaspoons avocado oil
- 1 large yellow onion, peeled and sliced thinly
- 1½ pounds 90% lean ground beef
- 2 teaspoons Worcestershire sauce
- 1 teaspoon dried minced onion
- 1 teaspoon sea salt
- ½ teaspoon ground black pepper
- 6 slices Swiss cheese

FOR SAUCE

- 3 tablespoons Tessemae's Unsweetened Ketchup
- 2 tablespoons Tessemae's Mayonnaise
- 2 teaspoons relish
- ¼ teaspoon Worcestershire sauce

1. To make Patty Melts: Heat oil in a large skillet over medium-high heat. Add onion and cook 15 minutes or until caramelized, stirring occasionally.
2. While onion is cooking, combine beef, Worcestershire, dried onion, salt, and pepper and mix well. Form beef mixture into six equal patties.
3. Transfer onion from skillet to a large plate and add patties to skillet. Cook 4 minutes on each side or until burgers reach desired level of doneness. Top each burger with 1 slice Swiss cheese and cover skillet to allow cheese to melt, about 2 minutes. Transfer burgers to each of six airtight containers.
4. To make Sauce: Add all ingredients to a small bowl and whisk until smooth. Top each burger with equal amounts Sauce. Cover and refrigerate until ready to eat, up to 1 week.
5. When ready to serve, transfer to a skillet over medium-low heat, cover, and cook 5 minutes or until heated through.

Spaghetti Squash Taco Bake

If you have some carbs to spare, you can make this recipe with your favorite macro-friendly pasta instead of spaghetti squash. Using a chickpea- or lentil-based pasta like Banza will also significantly increase the protein count.

SERVES 6

Per Serving:

Calories	327
Fat	13g
Sodium	753mg
Carbohydrates	28g
Fiber	7g
Sugar	8g
Protein	24g

2 teaspoons avocado oil

1 small yellow onion, peeled and diced

3 cloves garlic, peeled and minced

1 pound 93% lean ground turkey

1 (1.3-ounce) packet Siete Taco Seasoning

1 (15-ounce) can black beans, drained and rinsed

5 cups cooked spaghetti squash (1 large squash)

½ cup Siete Red Enchilada Sauce

1 cup shredded Mexican cheese blend

¼ cup chopped fresh cilantro

1. Preheat oven to 375°F.
2. Heat oil in a large skillet over medium-high heat. Add onion and cook 4 minutes. Add garlic and cook 1 minute. Crumble turkey into pan and cook 4 minutes, breaking up turkey with a spoon.
3. Sprinkle taco seasoning on top and continue cooking turkey until no longer pink, about 4 more minutes. Stir in beans and cook until heated through, about 2 minutes. Remove from heat and set aside.
4. Add squash to a 9" × 13" baking dish. Pour enchilada sauce on top and stir to combine. Spread out in an even layer and top with turkey mixture. Sprinkle cheese on top.
5. Bake 30 minutes or until casserole is bubbly and cheese is melted and starts to turn golden brown. Remove from oven and allow to cool 1 hour.
6. Divide evenly into six airtight containers and sprinkle cilantro on top. Cover and store in refrigerator up to 1 week, or in freezer up to 3 months, until ready to eat.
7. When ready to serve, transfer to a skillet over medium heat, cover, and cook 5 minutes or until heated through.

A TRICK TO CUTTING SPAGHETTI SQUASH

Spaghetti squash is notorious for being difficult to cut into, but here's a little trick: Pierce the squash in a few places with a knife, score it where you want to cut it, and then microwave it for about 3 minutes before cutting it with a sharp knife. This softens the squash and makes it easier to cut through.

Beef Bolognese

SERVES 6

Per Serving:

Calories	298
Fat	17g
Sodium	604mg
Carbohydrates	8g
Fiber	1g
Sugar	4g
Protein	26g

This isn't a traditional Bolognese, but it has a similar taste and comes together a lot more quickly. You can combine it with spaghetti squash or zucchini noodles or serve it on top of a scoop of cauliflower rice.

1 tablespoon extra-virgin olive oil
¼ cup minced celery
¼ cup minced yellow onion
3 cloves garlic, peeled and minced
1½ pounds 90% lean ground beef
¼ cup diced pancetta
2 cups no-sugar-added marinara sauce
¼ cup dry red wine
½ teaspoon red pepper flakes
½ teaspoon sea salt
¼ teaspoon onion powder

1. Heat oil in a large skillet over medium heat. Add celery and onion and cook 5 minutes or until celery starts to soften. Stir in garlic and cook 1 minute.
2. Crumble beef into pan and cook until no longer pink, about 8 minutes. Stir in remaining ingredients.
3. Reduce heat to low and simmer 1 hour. Remove from heat and allow to cool 1 hour.
4. Divide evenly into six airtight containers. Cover and store in refrigerator up to 1 week, or in freezer up to 3 months, until ready to eat.
5. When ready to serve, transfer to a saucepan over medium heat, cover, and cook 5 minutes or until heated through.

Mustard-Crusted Pork Tenderloin

If you're short on time or need to free up your oven for something else during meal prep, you can cook this pork in the slow cooker instead. Follow instructions as written, but add the pork to a slow cooker with a little bit of liquid—chicken broth works—and cook on high for 4 hours or low for 6–8 hours.

SERVES 6

Per Serving:

Calories	265
Fat	10g
Sodium	562mg
Carbohydrates	1g
Fiber	1g
Sugar	1g
Protein	41g

¾ cup Dijon mustard
2 teaspoons steak seasoning
1 teaspoon minced garlic
½ teaspoon dried rosemary
½ teaspoon sea salt
¼ teaspoon cracked black pepper
2 (1-pound) pork tenderloins

1. Preheat oven to 400°F. Line a baking sheet with parchment paper.
2. Combine all ingredients, except pork, in a small bowl. Spread mixture on pork and transfer coated pork to prepared baking sheet.
3. Roast 25 minutes or until internal temperature of pork reaches 155°F. Remove from oven and allow to rest 10 minutes.
4. Slice pork and divide pieces evenly into six airtight containers. Cover and store in refrigerator until ready to eat, up to 1 week.
5. When ready to serve, transfer to a skillet and cook over medium heat 5 minutes or until heated through.

Deconstructed Bacon Cheeseburgers

SERVES 6

Per Serving:

Calories	349
Fat	23g
Sodium	546mg
Carbohydrates	6g
Fiber	1g
Sugar	3g
Protein	27g

This recipe has all the taste of your favorite bacon cheeseburger but with considerably fewer carbs and none of the artificial ingredients that come with the drive-through. If you want to add some crunch and you have carbs to spare, you can crush some plantain chips on top right before eating.

⅓ cup Tessemae's Unsweetened Ketchup

¼ cup Tessemae's Mayonnaise

2 tablespoons sweet relish

1 teaspoon avocado oil

⅓ cup minced yellow onion

1½ pounds 90% lean ground beef

2 teaspoons steak seasoning

1 teaspoon sea salt

¾ cup shredded Cheddar cheese

6 tablespoons crumbled cooked no-sugar-added bacon

¾ cup finely diced Roma tomato

6 cups chopped iceberg lettuce

1. Add ketchup, mayo, and relish to a small bowl and whisk until smooth. Set aside.
2. Heat oil in a large skillet over medium heat. Add onion and cook 4 minutes. Crumble beef into skillet and cook 4 minutes. Sprinkle steak seasoning and salt on beef and continue cooking 4 minutes or until no longer pink. Remove beef from heat and allow to cool, about 15 minutes.
3. Scoop 2 tablespoons ketchup mixture into each of six quart-sized Mason jars. Top each with equal parts beef, 2 tablespoons cheese, 1 tablespoon crumbled bacon, 2 tablespoons tomato, and 1 cup lettuce. Cover and store in refrigerator until ready to eat, up to 1 week.
4. When ready to serve, shake vigorously.

Blue Cheese Spinach Burgers

If you're not a fan of the strong flavor of blue cheese, you can swap it out for feta cheese or even shredded mozzarella. Just keep in mind that this will slightly change the macros.

SERVES 6

Per Serving:

Calories	218
Fat	13g
Sodium	537mg
Carbohydrates	1g
Fiber	0g
Sugar	0g
Protein	24g

¾ cup chopped fresh spinach
4 cloves garlic, peeled and minced
2 teaspoons dried minced onion
1 teaspoon sea salt
½ teaspoon ground black pepper
¼ cup crumbled blue cheese
1½ pounds 90% lean ground beef

1. Preheat grill to medium-high heat.
2. Combine all ingredients in a large bowl. Divide into six equal portions and form into patties.
3. Place patties on grill and cook 8 minutes (or until burgers reach desired level of doneness), flipping once while cooking. Allow to rest 2 minutes.
4. Store each burger in a separate airtight container in refrigerator until ready to eat, up to 1 week.
5. When ready to serve, transfer to a skillet, cover, and cook over medium heat 5 minutes or until heated through.

FREEZE FOR LATER

Rather than cooking these burgers for the week, you can stock your freezer with uncooked patties that you can prepare in minutes for a quick meal. After you form the beef mixture into patties, lay them out on a parchment paper–lined baking sheet and freeze them for 1 hour. Stack them, with a piece of parchment paper in between each patty, then transfer them to a gallon-sized freezer bag and store in the freezer for up to 3 months. When you're ready to eat, you can throw one right on the grill without defrosting.

Beef Tamale Casserole

SERVES 6

Per Serving:

Calories	342
Fat	16g
Sodium	600mg
Carbohydrates	19g
Fiber	2g
Sugar	4g
Protein	28g

You can play around with the macros in this recipe by using beef with different fat content or swapping it out for shredded chicken or ground turkey instead. Omitting the corn will lower the carbs, and reducing the cheese will lower the fat.

1½ pounds 90% lean ground beef
1 (1.3-ounce) packet Siete Taco Seasoning
1 (14-ounce) can sweet corn kernels, drained
1 (4-ounce) can fire-roasted diced green chiles, drained
⅔ cup Siete Red Enchilada Sauce
¾ cup shredded Mexican cheese blend

1. Heat a large skillet over medium-high heat. Crumble beef into skillet and cook 4 minutes. Add taco seasoning and continue cooking until beef is no longer pink, about 4 more minutes. Transfer beef to a 9" × 13" baking dish.
2. Combine corn and green chiles in a medium bowl and pour over beef. Pour enchilada sauce over corn mixture. Scatter cheese evenly over top of sauce.
3. Bake 20 minutes or until casserole is bubbly and cheese is slightly browned. Remove from oven and allow to cool 1 hour.
4. Divide evenly into six airtight containers. Cover and store in refrigerator up to 1 week, or in freezer up to 3 months, until ready to eat.
5. When ready to serve, transfer to a skillet, cover, and cook over medium heat 5 minutes or until heated through.

Baked Taquitos

When you're ready to eat these taquitos, consider heating them in an air fryer for a few minutes to crisp them back up instead of broiling.

SERVES 8

Per Serving (2 taquitos):

Calories	222
Fat	10g
Sodium	470mg
Carbohydrates	17g
Fiber	2g
Sugar	1g
Protein	16g

- 1 teaspoon extra-virgin olive oil
- 1 small yellow onion, peeled and diced
- 2 cloves garlic, peeled and minced
- 1 pound 90% lean ground beef
- 2 teaspoons chili powder
- 1 teaspoon ground cumin
- ½ teaspoon dried oregano
- ½ teaspoon paprika
- 1 teaspoon sea salt
- ½ teaspoon ground black pepper
- ⅛ teaspoon red pepper flakes
- ½ cup Siete Red Enchilada Sauce
- 1 cup shredded Mexican cheese blend
- 16 (4.5") corn tortillas

1. Preheat oven to 425°F. Line a baking sheet with parchment paper.
2. Heat oil in a large skillet over medium-high heat. Add onion and cook 3 minutes or until translucent. Add garlic and cook another 1 minute.
3. Crumble beef into pan and cook 4 minutes or until it starts to brown. Mix chili powder, cumin, oregano, paprika, salt, black pepper, and red pepper flakes in a small bowl. Sprinkle over beef and continue cooking until no longer pink, about 4 more minutes.
4. Stir in enchilada sauce. Remove from heat and add cheese, stirring until melted.
5. Wet two paper towels and squeeze out excess water. Put 2 tortillas between damp paper towels and microwave 30 seconds. Repeat with remaining tortillas.
6. Lay tortillas flat and fill each with 1 heaping tablespoon beef mixture. Tightly roll up tortillas and place, seam-side down, on prepared baking sheet.
7. Bake 15 minutes or until taquitos are crispy and turning golden brown. Remove from oven and allow to cool 30 minutes.
8. Transfer 2 taquitos to each of eight airtight containers. Cover and store in refrigerator up to 1 week, or in freezer up to 3 months, until ready to eat.
9. When ready to serve, transfer to a baking sheet and broil under low heat 3 minutes or until heated through and crispy.

Instant Pot® Beef Gyros

SERVES 6

Per Serving:

Calories	262
Fat	12g
Sodium	638mg
Carbohydrates	4g
Fiber	1g
Sugar	3g
Protein	35g

On their own, these Instant Pot® Beef Gyros are low in carbs, but you can serve them with a warm pita or in a lavash wrap—whatever choice fits in your macro allowance (and with your lifestyle). If you have chopped lettuce, tomatoes, or red onions on hand, you can add them as toppings before serving.

FOR BEEF

⅓ cup beef broth

2 pounds beef chuck roast

1 large white onion, peeled and thinly sliced

2 tablespoons lemon juice

1 tablespoon avocado oil

2 teaspoons garlic powder

2 teaspoons dried oregano

1 teaspoon sea salt

½ teaspoon ground black pepper

FOR TZATZIKI SAUCE

1 cup 2% plain Greek yogurt

1 cup shredded cucumber

2 teaspoons dried dill

½ teaspoon sea salt

3 cloves garlic, peeled and minced

1 teaspoon lemon juice

1. To make Beef: Pour broth into Instant Pot®. Place chuck roast in pot and top with onion.
2. In a small bowl, whisk together lemon juice, oil, garlic powder, oregano, salt, and pepper. Pour over roast. Close the lid, set to manual/high pressure, and set time for 40 minutes. When time is up, allow pressure to release naturally.
3. Open lid and remove beef. Shred with two forks and divide mixture evenly into six airtight containers.
4. To make Tzatziki Sauce: Combine yogurt and cucumber in a small bowl. Stir in dill, salt, and garlic until smooth. Stir in lemon juice. Pour equal amounts of Sauce into each container of Beef.
5. Cover and store in refrigerator until ready to eat, up to 1 week.
6. When ready to serve, transfer to a skillet, cover, and cook over medium heat 5 minutes or until heated through.

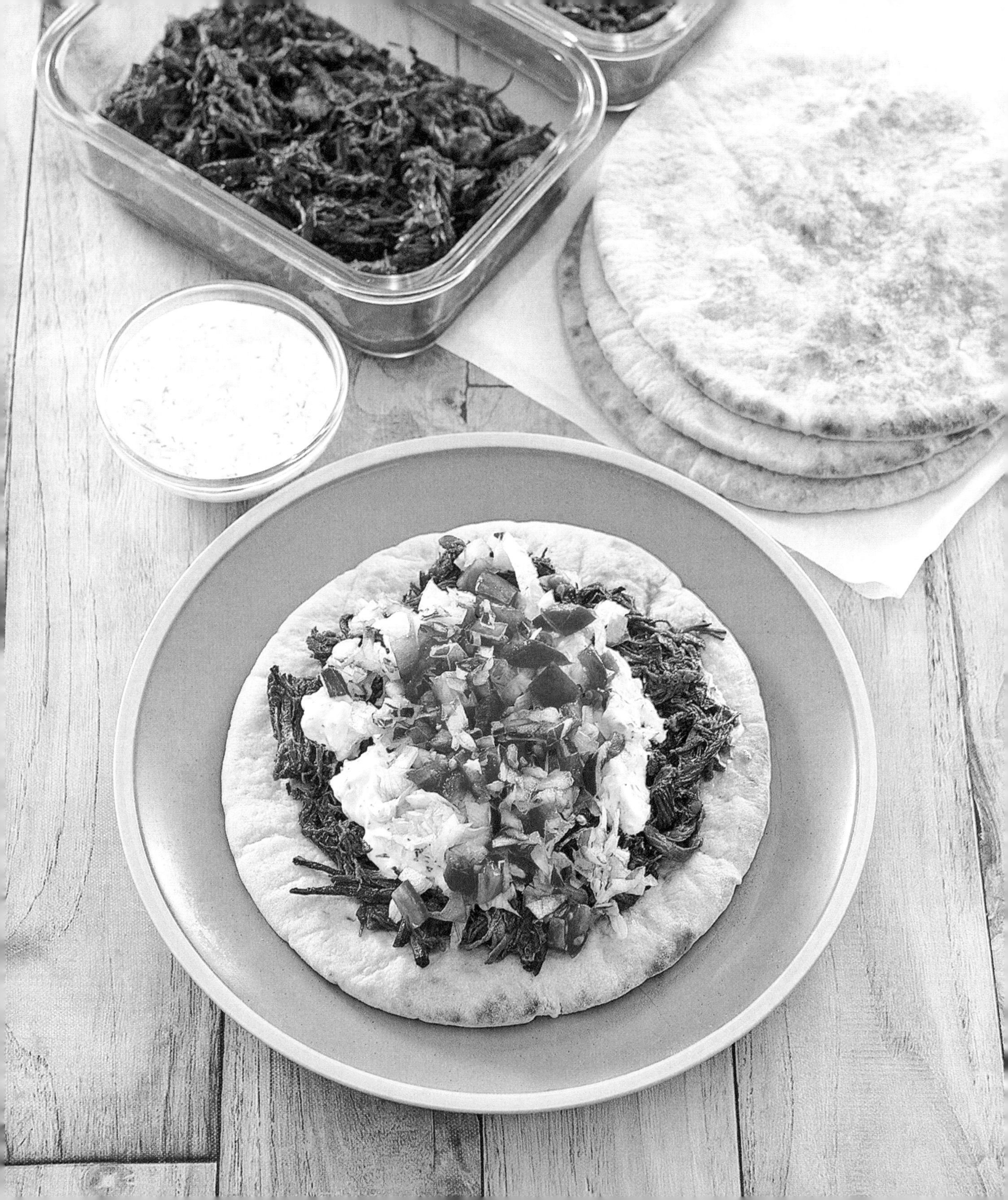

One-Pot Beef and Zucchini Skillet

SERVES 6

Per Serving:

Calories	228
Fat	13g
Sodium	479mg
Carbohydrates	2g
Fiber	1g
Sugar	1g
Protein	24g

This easy weeknight meal can be made in huge batches and stored for later. It's also fully customizable and an excellent way to use whatever is leftover in your refrigerator. You can follow the same steps using different meats and vegetable combinations. Just make sure to recalculate the macros accordingly!

2 teaspoons avocado oil

1½ pounds 90% lean ground beef

2 teaspoons steak seasoning

1 teaspoon garlic powder

2 small zucchini, seeded and diced

1 (10-ounce) package frozen cauliflower rice

1 teaspoon sea salt

½ teaspoon ground black pepper

1. Heat oil in a large skillet over medium-high heat. Crumble beef into pan and cook 4 minutes or until it starts to brown. Stir in steak seasoning and garlic powder and cook 2 minutes.
2. Add zucchini and cauliflower rice, cover, and cook 5 minutes or until vegetables are softened. Stir in salt and pepper. Remove from heat and allow to cool 30 minutes.
3. Divide evenly into six airtight containers. Store in refrigerator up to 1 week, or in freezer up to 3 months, until ready to eat.
4. When ready to serve, transfer to a skillet, cover, and cook over medium heat 5 minutes or until heated through.

HOMEMADE STEAK SEASONING

You can use any steak seasoning that fits into your macros and has a good ingredient list, but if you want to make a delicious (and quick) version at home, combine 2 tablespoons paprika, 2 tablespoons salt, 2 tablespoons ground black pepper, 1 tablespoon granulated garlic, 1 tablespoon granulated onion, 1 tablespoon ground coriander, 1 tablespoon dried dill, and 2 teaspoons red pepper flakes. Use what you need and store the rest in an airtight container in your pantry.

Mongolian Beef and Broccoli

Depending on your macro allowance, you can serve this Mongolian Beef and Broccoli with cauliflower rice or regular brown or white rice. It's also delicious on top of a baked potato or quinoa or served on its own.

SERVES 6

Per Serving:

Calories	235
Fat	10g
Sodium	314mg
Carbohydrates	14g
Fiber	1g
Sugar	3g
Protein	24g

2 teaspoons avocado oil, divided

3 cloves garlic, peeled and minced

1 teaspoon grated fresh ginger

⅓ cup coconut aminos

¼ cup beef broth

⅓ cup Swerve brown sweetener

1½ pounds flank steak, cut into ¼" slices

2 cups broccoli florets

2 tablespoons sesame seeds

¼ cup chopped scallions

1. Heat 1 teaspoon oil in a small saucepan over medium heat. Add garlic and ginger and cook 1 minute. Stir in coconut aminos, beef broth, and brown sweetener. Bring to a gentle boil and boil 5 minutes.
2. While sauce is cooking, heat remaining 1 teaspoon oil in a large skillet over medium-high heat. Add steak and cook 3 minutes, browning both sides. Add broccoli and cook 1 minute.
3. Pour sauce over steak and broccoli and reduce heat to medium-low. Cook another 4 minutes or until steak is cooked through and sauce is thickened. Remove from heat and sprinkle sesame seeds and scallions on top. Allow to cool 30 minutes.
4. Divide evenly into six airtight containers. Store in refrigerator until ready to eat, up to 1 week.
5. When ready to serve, transfer to a skillet, cover, and cook over medium heat 5 minutes or until heated through.

WHITE VERSUS BROWN RICE

When it comes to macros, white rice and brown rice are pretty similar. One cup of cooked white rice has 45 grams of carbohydrates, 4.3 grams of protein, and 0.4 grams of fat. The same serving of brown rice has 46 grams of carbohydrates, 4.5 grams of protein, and 1.6 grams of fat. While you'll add a gram of fat if you go with the brown rice, you'll also be getting more fiber. There's 3.5 grams in brown rice and just 0.6 grams in white rice.

Pecan-Crusted Pork Chops

SERVES 6

Per Serving:

Calories	465
Fat	33g
Sodium	186mg
Carbohydrates	8g
Fiber	5g
Sugar	3g
Protein	32g

Pecans are packed with protein, but they're also pretty high in fat. Because of this, you may need to work these Pecan-Crusted Pork Chops into your meal plan with other lower-fat dishes. If you want to reduce the fat content, you can use fewer pecans and just coat the chops a little more lightly.

2 cups whole pecans

½ teaspoon ground cinnamon

⅛ teaspoon sea salt

3 tablespoons Tessemae's Honey Mustard

6 (4-ounce) boneless pork chops

2 tablespoons extra-virgin olive oil

2 tablespoons ChocZero Maple-Flavored Syrup

1. Preheat oven to 350°F.
2. Add pecans, cinnamon, and salt to a food processor. Pulse until large crumbs form, about 20 seconds. Transfer to a shallow dish.
3. Spread honey mustard evenly on both sides of each pork chop. Press pork chops into pecan mixture, coating both sides.
4. Heat oil in a large skillet over medium heat. Add pork chops and sear 2 minutes on each side.
5. Transfer pork chops to an ungreased 9" × 13" baking dish and bake 15 minutes or until pork chops reach an internal temperature of 165°F. Remove from oven and drizzle maple syrup on top. Allow to cool 30 minutes.
6. Place 1 pork chop in each of six airtight containers. Cover and store in refrigerator until ready to eat, up to 1 week.
7. When ready to serve, reheat in a skillet 5 minutes on low to avoid burning pecan crust.

Sesame Pork Tenderloin

ChocZero Maple-Flavored Syrup is a low-glycemic sweetener that's made without sugar and sugar alcohols. While the label says it has 16 grams of carbs per serving, 15 grams come from fiber. This means it has just 1 gram of net carbs, the only type of carb that affects your blood sugar.

SERVES 6

Per Serving:

Calories	192
Fat	4g
Sodium	579mg
Carbohydrates	19g
Fiber	19g
Sugar	2g
Protein	22g

FOR PORK

- 1½ pounds pork tenderloin, cut into 3" strips
- 2 teaspoons toasted sesame oil
- 1 teaspoon garlic powder
- 1 teaspoon sea salt
- ½ teaspoon ground black pepper
- ½ teaspoon ground ginger

FOR SAUCE

- ½ cup ChocZero Maple-Flavored Syrup
- 3 tablespoons lime juice
- 2 tablespoons sriracha
- 1 tablespoon coconut aminos
- 4 cloves garlic, peeled and minced
- 1 tablespoon sesame seeds

1. To make Pork: Place pork in a large bowl. Drizzle oil on top and toss to coat. Sprinkle garlic powder, salt, pepper, and ginger on pork, coating all sides as evenly as possible.
2. Heat a large skillet over medium-high heat. Add coated pork and cook 7 minutes or until pork is no longer pink, stirring frequently.
3. To make Sauce: While pork is cooking, add maple syrup, lime juice, sriracha, coconut aminos, and garlic to a medium bowl and whisk until smooth.
4. Pour Sauce over Pork and stir to coat. Cook another 2 minutes or until Sauce starts to thicken. Sprinkle sesame seeds on top.
5. Divide evenly into six airtight containers. Cover and store in refrigerator up to 1 week, or in freezer up to 3 months, until ready to eat.
6. When ready to serve, transfer to a skillet, cover, and cook over medium-low heat for 5 minutes or until heated through.

NET CARBS VERSUS TOTAL CARBS

Generally, macro counting focuses on total carbs rather than net carbs, but if you want to get a little more specific, you might want to pay attention to net carbs. Net carbs are the carbohydrates that your body can digest and use. Some carbs, like fiber and sugar alcohols, pass through your digestive system untouched so they don't have an impact on your blood sugar. To calculate net carbs, simply take the total carbohydrates and subtract the fiber and sugar alcohols.

Pork and Broccolini Stir-Fry

SERVES 6

Per Serving:

Calories	184
Fat	6g
Sodium	786mg
Carbohydrates	5g
Fiber	1g
Sugar	2g
Protein	27g

If you want to add some crunch to this stir-fry, you can stir in some crushed peanuts after everything is done cooking or sprinkle them on top before eating. If you have some carbs to spare, serve on top of cooked rice noodles. If you don't, it's delicious as is or over cauliflower rice.

FOR SAUCE

3 cloves garlic, peeled and minced
2 tablespoons coconut aminos
2 tablespoons Swerve granular sweetener
2 tablespoons fish sauce
1 teaspoon red curry paste
1 teaspoon minced fresh ginger
½ teaspoon ground coriander
½ teaspoon sea salt
¼ teaspoon ground black pepper
¼ teaspoon red pepper flakes

FOR PORK

1 tablespoon toasted sesame oil
1½ pounds pork tenderloin, cut into 3" strips
½ teaspoon sea salt
½ teaspoon ground black pepper
2 small shallots, peeled and minced
1 pound broccolini stalks, chopped
2 teaspoons fresh lime juice
1 Thai red pepper, sliced

1. To make Sauce: Add all sauce ingredients to a medium bowl and whisk until smooth. Set aside.
2. To make Pork: Heat oil in a large skillet or wok over medium-high heat. Add pork and sprinkle with salt and pepper. Cook 2 minutes, then add shallots and cook 2 more minutes. Add broccolini and continue cooking 4 minutes or until tender.
3. Pour Sauce over Pork and vegetables and stir. Add lime juice and Thai pepper and cook 3 more minutes or until sauce is bubbly and starts to thicken. Remove from heat and allow to cool 30 minutes.
4. Divide evenly into six airtight containers. Cover and store in refrigerator until ready to eat, up to 1 week.
5. When ready to serve, transfer to a skillet, cover, and cook over medium-low heat 5 minutes or until heated through.

Chili Beef and Rice

This recipe calls for Yai's Thai Sweet Chili Sauce, which is considerably lower in carbs than other chili sauces, since it's sweetened with natural fruit juices instead of added sugar. If you use a different sauce, it will change the carbs significantly, so keep that in mind when prepping.

SERVES 6

Per Serving:

Calories	328
Fat	13g
Sodium	316mg
Carbohydrates	26g
Fiber	4g
Sugar	4g
Protein	26g

2 teaspoons extra-virgin olive oil

1½ pounds 90% lean ground beef

1 teaspoon chili powder

½ teaspoon sea salt

¼ teaspoon ground black pepper

1 pound Brussels sprouts, trimmed and quartered

⅓ cup Yai's Thai Sweet Chili Sauce

3 cups cooked brown rice

1. Heat oil in a large skillet over medium heat. Crumble beef into pan and cook 2 minutes. Sprinkle chili powder, salt, and pepper on top and stir to incorporate.
2. Add Brussels sprouts and stir. Cover and cook 6 minutes or until beef is cooked through and Brussels sprouts are tender. Pour chili sauce on top and stir to combine. Cook 1 more minute or until heated through. Remove from heat and allow to cool 30 minutes.
3. Scoop ½ cup brown rice into each of six airtight containers. Top with equal portions beef and Brussels sprouts mixture. Cover and store in refrigerator until ready to eat, up to 1 week.
4. When ready to serve, transfer to a skillet, cover, and cook over medium heat 5 minutes or until heated through.

Barbecue Pork Tenderloin

SERVES 6

Per Serving:

Calories	180
Fat	4g
Sodium	993mg
Carbohydrates	13g
Fiber	4g
Sugar	9g
Protein	23g

MAKING YOUR OWN BARBECUE SAUCE

If you can't find any no-sugar-added versions at the grocery store, you can easily make your own. Combine 1½ cups Lakanto Golden Monkfruit Sweetener, 1½ cups no-sugar-added ketchup, ½ cup red wine vinegar, ½ cup water, 1 tablespoon Worcestershire sauce, 2½ tablespoons dry mustard, 2 teaspoons paprika, 2 teaspoons sea salt, 1½ teaspoons ground black pepper, and 1 teaspoon hot sauce in a blender and blend until smooth.

Many commercial barbecue sauces have added sugar, which significantly increases their carb count. If you don't have Primal Kitchen Classic BBQ Sauce, make sure you're using another sauce without any added sugar.

1 teaspoon granulated garlic
1 teaspoon granulated onion
1 teaspoon sea salt
½ teaspoon ground black pepper
1 (1½-pound) pork tenderloin
3 cups Primal Kitchen Classic BBQ Sauce, divided

1. Sprinkle garlic, onion, salt, and pepper on pork and place in a slow cooker. Pour 2 cups barbecue sauce over pork.
2. Cover and cook 8 hours on low or until pork is tender and falls apart easily with a fork. Use two forks to shred pork and stir into barbecue sauce.
3. Stir remaining 1 cup barbecue sauce into slow cooker, cover, and cook 30 more minutes. Allow to cool 1 hour.
4. Divide evenly into six airtight containers. Cover and store in refrigerator until ready to eat, up to 1 week.
5. When ready to serve, transfer to a skillet, cover, and cook over medium heat 5 minutes or until heated through.

Garlic Butter Steak with Zucchini Noodles

There's no need to cook these zucchini noodles before adding them to your meal prep container. As the steak sits on top of the raw zucchini noodles, they will soften and take on the flavors of the garlic butter.

SERVES 6

Per Serving:

Calories	280
Fat	18g
Sodium	466mg
Carbohydrates	4g
Fiber	2g
Sugar	4g
Protein	25g

1 tablespoon avocado oil

3 tablespoons unsalted grass-fed butter, softened

2 teaspoons minced garlic

2 teaspoons chopped fresh parsley

1 teaspoon sea salt

½ teaspoon ground black pepper

6 (4-ounce) sirloin steaks

3 large zucchini, spiralized

1. Preheat grill to high heat. Brush oil on grill grate.
2. Combine butter, garlic, and parsley in a small bowl. Set aside.
3. Sprinkle salt and pepper on each side of steaks. Place steak on grill and cook 5 minutes per side or until steak reaches desired level of doneness.
4. Remove steaks from grill and brush each with equal parts butter mixture.
5. Divide zucchini noodles evenly into six airtight containers. Put one steak on top of each. Cover and store in refrigerator until ready to eat, up to 1 week.
6. When ready to serve, transfer to a skillet and cook over medium-low heat, flipping once, 5 minutes or until heated through.

Gouda-Stuffed Pork Chops

SERVES 6

Per Serving:

Calories	263
Fat	15g
Sodium	912mg
Carbohydrates	0g
Fiber	0g
Sugar	1g
Protein	32g

If smoked Gouda is a little too strong for your tastes, you can go with smoked mozzarella or smoked Cheddar. These varieties are easy to find at most grocery stores, and they melt similarly to each other and have similar macros. Plus, the smoky flavor really adds a little something special to the dish.

6 (4-ounce) boneless pork chops

1½ teaspoons sea salt, divided

1 teaspoon ground black pepper, divided

½ teaspoon garlic powder

½ teaspoon ground sage

¾ cup shredded smoked Gouda cheese

6 tablespoons chopped fresh parsley

2 teaspoons avocado oil

1. Preheat oven to 400°F. Line a baking sheet with parchment paper.
2. Using a kitchen mallet, pound pork chops to ¼" thickness. Sprinkle ½ teaspoon salt, ½ teaspoon pepper, garlic powder, and sage on one side of each pork chop.
3. Sprinkle 2 tablespoons cheese and 1 tablespoon parsley on seasoned side of each pork chop. Carefully roll up each pork chop and secure with kitchen twine or a couple toothpicks. Transfer to prepared baking sheet, then drizzle oil on top and sprinkle with remaining 1 teaspoon salt and ½ teaspoon pepper.
4. Bake 20 minutes or until pork is cooked through and cheese is melted and bubbly. Allow to cool 30 minutes.
5. Transfer the pork chops to each of six airtight containers. Cover and store in refrigerator until ready to eat, up to 1 week.
6. When ready to serve, transfer to a skillet, cover, and cook over medium-low heat 5 minutes or until heated through.

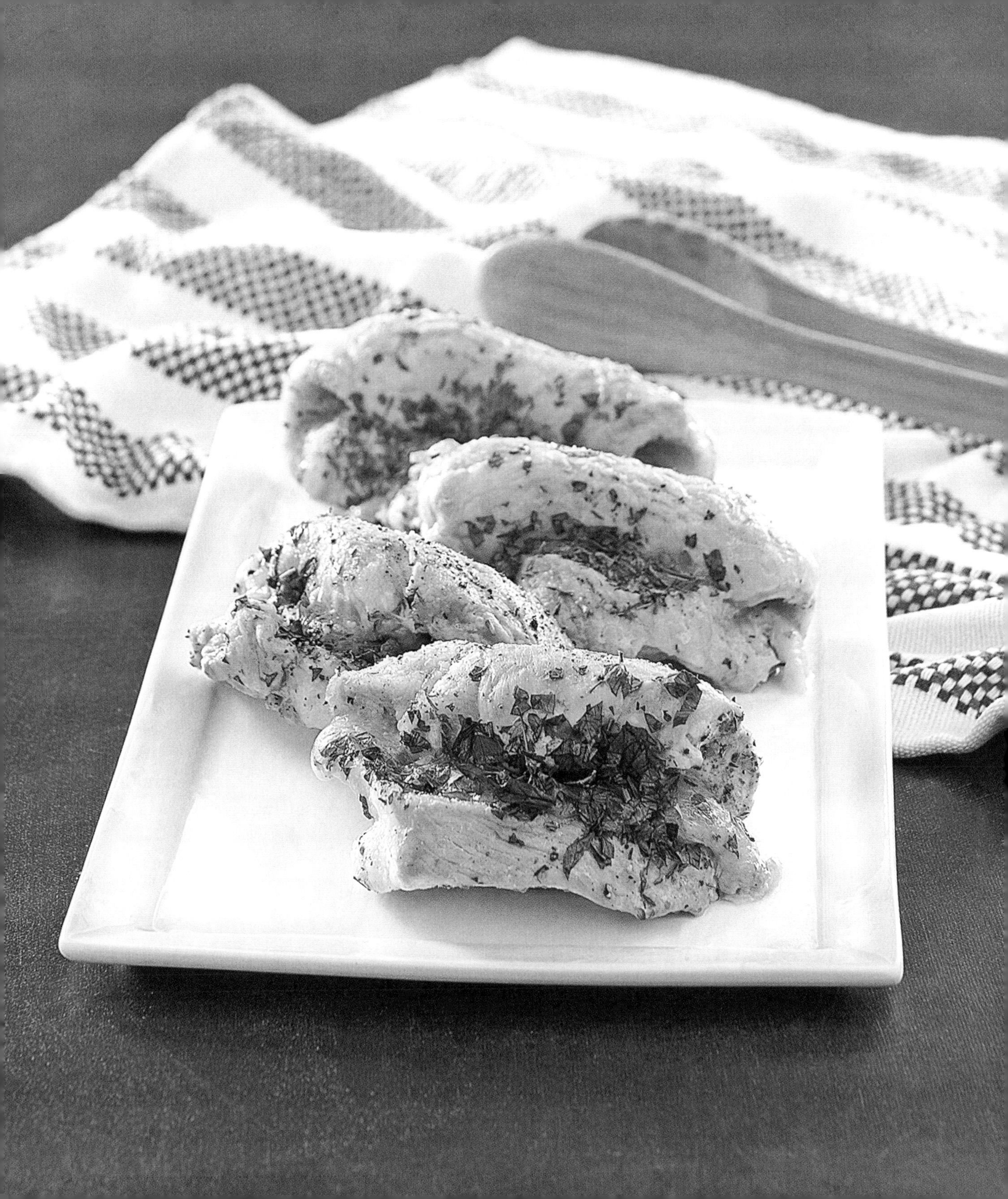

Sesame Ginger Ground Beef Skillet

SERVES 6

Per Serving:

Calories	253
Fat	14g
Sodium	322mg
Carbohydrates	6g
Fiber	1g
Sugar	4g
Protein	24g

This hearty dish is a great protein source for power bowls or as a protein-packed ingredient in Mason jar salads. You can also serve it with cauliflower rice or regular rice, on top of a baked potato, or with a side of mashed cauliflower or potatoes, depending on your carb allowance.

1½ pounds 90% lean ground beef
⅓ cup coconut aminos
¼ cup no-sugar-added beef broth
1 teaspoon toasted sesame oil
1 tablespoon Swerve granular sweetener
1 tablespoon minced fresh ginger
3 cloves garlic, peeled and minced
2 cups sliced white mushrooms
1 cup frozen peas
2 tablespoons sesame seeds

1. Crumble ground beef into a large skillet over medium-high heat. Add coconut aminos, broth, oil, sweetener, ginger, and garlic to a medium bowl and whisk until smooth. Pour over beef and cook 5 minutes or until beef starts to brown and sauce starts to thicken.
2. Stir in mushrooms and cook 4 minutes or until mushrooms are tender. Stir in peas and cook 1 more minute. Sprinkle sesame seeds on top. Remove from heat and allow to cool 30 minutes.
3. Divide evenly into six airtight containers. Cover and store in refrigerator until ready to eat, up to 1 week.
4. When ready to serve, transfer to a skillet, cover, and cook over medium heat 5 minutes or until heated through.

CHAPTER 7

Seafood Main Meals

Garlic Shrimp with Zucchini and Peppers

SERVES 4

Per Serving:

Calories	158
Fat	7g
Sodium	707mg
Carbohydrates	6g
Fiber	3g
Sugar	4g
Protein	17g

THE BENEFITS OF GRASS-FED BUTTER

Butter made with the milk of grass-fed cows is higher in certain nutrients, like vitamin A and conjugated linoleic acid (CLA), than its conventional counterpart. CLA has been shown to support the immune system, strengthen bones, and help balance your blood sugar. Some studies also show that it can help improve body composition, meaning it can reduce body fat and help you maintain a healthy body weight.

You don't have to cook the zucchini in this recipe. It will soften as it sits in the sauce in the refrigerator and a bit more when you reheat your meal, getting to the perfect consistency.

3 medium zucchini, spiralized

2 teaspoons extra-virgin olive oil

1 tablespoon unsalted grass-fed butter

1 large red bell pepper, seeded and sliced thinly

4 cloves garlic, peeled and minced

2 tablespoons lemon juice

¼ cup chicken broth

1 pound raw medium shrimp, peeled and deveined

1 teaspoon Italian seasoning

¼ teaspoon sea salt

¼ teaspoon ground black pepper

⅛ teaspoon red pepper flakes

1. Divide zucchini noodles into four airtight containers. Set aside.
2. Heat oil and butter in a large skillet over medium-high heat. Add bell pepper and cook 5 minutes. Stir in garlic and cook another 1 minute. Pour in lemon juice and broth and stir.
3. Add shrimp to skillet and toss to coat with butter mixture. Sprinkle Italian seasoning, salt, black pepper, and red pepper flakes on shrimp. Cook 2 minutes, flip over, and cook another 2 minutes or until shrimp is cooked through.
4. Put equal amounts of shrimp on top of zucchini in each container. Scoop equal amounts of sauce on top. Cover and store in refrigerator until ready to eat, up to 4 days.
5. When ready to serve, transfer to a skillet, cover, and cook over low heat 5 minutes or until heated through.

Tuna Zucchini Cakes

The gluten-free rolled oats in this recipe help hold the cakes together, but if you want to lower the carbs, you can omit them—just be careful when you're cooking and flipping them so they don't crumble.

SERVES 4

Per Serving (2 cakes):

Calories	274
Fat	11g
Sodium	1,148mg
Carbohydrates	11g
Fiber	3g
Sugar	5g
Protein	33g

FOR CAKES

- 2 large zucchini, grated
- ½ teaspoon sea salt
- 2 (5-ounce) cans solid white albacore tuna packed in water, drained
- ½ cup gluten-free rolled oats
- ½ cup shredded mozzarella cheese
- 3 large eggs, lightly beaten
- 1 teaspoon garlic salt
- 1 teaspoon onion powder
- ½ teaspoon dried dill
- ½ teaspoon ground black pepper
- 2 teaspoons avocado oil

FOR SAUCE

- ½ cup 2% plain Greek yogurt
- 1 tablespoon lemon juice
- 1 teaspoon garlic salt
- ¾ teaspoon dried dill
- ½ teaspoon ground cumin
- 1 tablespoon seeded minced jalapeño

1. To make Cakes: Put zucchini in a strainer and sprinkle with salt. Let sweat 10 minutes, then transfer to a cheesecloth or nut bag and squeeze out all excess liquid. Transfer zucchini to a large mixing bowl.
2. Add remaining ingredients, except oil, and mix well. Divide mixture into eight equal portions and shape each portion into a patty.
3. Heat oil in a large skillet over medium-high heat. Add patties and cook 3 minutes on each side or until browned and crispy on the outside. Transfer to a paper towel–lined plate.
4. Allow to cool 30 minutes.
5. To make Sauce: While Cakes are cooling, whisk all ingredients in a small bowl until smooth.
6. Place two Cakes in each of four airtight containers. Scoop 2 tablespoons Sauce on top of Cakes. Cover and store in refrigerator until ready to eat, up to 1 week.
7. Serve cold.

Goddess Grain Bowl with Shrimp

SERVES 4

Per Serving:

Calories	482
Fat	22g
Sodium	323mg
Carbohydrates	36g
Fiber	1g
Sugar	6g
Protein	37g

Shrimp is a great protein source for this grain bowl, but you can swap it out for other meats if you don't like shrimp or just want to switch things up.

3 cups cooked sprouted quinoa

1 pound cooked peeled deveined small shrimp

½ cup diced cucumber

1 cup edamame beans

1 cup sliced green bell pepper

1 cup broccoli sprouts

½ cup Tessemae's Green Goddess Dressing and Marinade

1. Scoop ¾ cup quinoa into each of four airtight containers. Add equal parts shrimp, 2 tablespoons cucumber, ¼ cup edamame, ¼ cup green pepper, and ¼ cup broccoli sprouts to each container.
2. Pour 2 tablespoons dressing into each of four small containers. Place small containers in large containers, cover, and store in refrigerator until ready to eat, up to 4 days.
3. Serve cold.

Shrimp Chowder

If you want to cut the carbs in this chowder, you can replace the potatoes with cauliflower or turnips, which have a similar taste and texture. You can also play around with different types of milk or cream to adjust the fat content to your needs.

SERVES 4

Per Serving:

Calories	357
Fat	16g
Sodium	1,086mg
Carbohydrates	27g
Fiber	3g
Sugar	3g
Protein	27g

2 tablespoons Nutiva Buttery Flavor Coconut Oil

2 large shallots, peeled and minced

1 cup sliced celery

3 cloves garlic, peeled and minced

½ teaspoon ground fennel

½ teaspoon dried thyme

½ teaspoon smoked paprika

⅓ cup dry white wine

3 cups chicken broth

1 teaspoon fish sauce

1 teaspoon sea salt

2 cups peeled diced yellow potatoes

2 cups light coconut milk

1 pound raw peeled deveined small shrimp

1. Heat oil in a large stockpot or Dutch oven over medium heat. Add shallots and celery and cook until celery starts to soften, about 5 minutes. Stir in garlic and cook another 1 minute. Sprinkle fennel, thyme, and paprika over mixture and cook 2 more minutes.
2. Add wine to skillet and cook 3 minutes or until some liquid evaporates. Stir in broth, fish sauce, and salt. Add potatoes, raise the heat to high, and bring to a boil. Reduce the heat to low and simmer 10 minutes or until potatoes are tender.
3. Stir in coconut milk and shrimp and cook 2 minutes. Remove from heat and allow shrimp to continue cooking in skillet 5 more minutes.
4. Transfer equal amounts of chowder to each of four airtight containers. Cover and store in refrigerator up to 4 days, or in freezer up to 3 months, until ready to eat.
5. When ready to serve, transfer to a saucepan, cover, and cook over low heat 5 minutes or until heated through.

LIGHT VERSUS FULL-FAT COCONUT MILK

Real coconut milk is naturally high in fat, but you can still benefit from the creaminess of the ingredient by choosing the light version. Light coconut milk refers to canned coconut milk, of which there are usually two options available. The full-fat canned coconut milk includes coconut milk and cream, which is where most of the fat is contained. Light coconut milk contains coconut milk mixed with a bit of water. If you only have full-fat coconut milk, you can mix it 1:1 with water to get the same effect.

Oven-Roasted Mackerel

SERVES 4

Per Serving:

Calories	210
Fat	13g
Sodium	645mg
Carbohydrates	0g
Fiber	0g
Sugar	0g
Protein	23g

A RARE SOURCE OF VITAMIN D

Mackerel is one of just a handful of foods that are naturally high in vitamin D. A 4-ounce serving of mackerel contains around 19.6 micrograms of vitamin D, which converts to 784 international units (IU)—more than the National Institutes of Health recommends that you get in a day. Vitamin D not only contributes to strong bones and teeth; it also supports your immune system and improves your mental health.

Salmon gets a lot of love for its omega-3 fatty acid content, but mackerel is another excellent option that's also low in mercury and high in vitamin D. If you're new to mackerel, give it a shot—you'll be pleasantly surprised.

4 (4-ounce) Spanish mackerel fillets

2 tablespoons extra-virgin olive oil

1 teaspoon minced garlic

1 teaspoon ground cumin

¾ teaspoon paprika

½ teaspoon ground coriander

1 teaspoon sea salt

½ teaspoon ground black pepper

8 slices lemon

1. Preheat oven to 350°F. Lay out four pieces of aluminum foil.
2. Place 1 mackerel fillet on each piece of foil. Brush oil on top of each fillet, add ¼ teaspoon garlic on top, then sprinkle evenly with spices. Top each fillet with 2 lemon slices.
3. Wrap up each fillet in foil, then place the foil packets on a baking sheet. Bake 30 minutes or until fish flakes apart easily with a fork. Remove from oven and allow to cool 20 minutes.
4. Open foil packets and transfer fillets to each of four airtight containers. Cover and store in refrigerator until ready to eat, up to 4 days.
5. When ready to serve, transfer to a skillet, cover, and cook over low heat 5 minutes or until heated through.

Broiled Salmon with Cabbage

Cabbage is an under-utilized and under-appreciated vegetable, but it's an excellent low-carb vegetable that adds a lot of flavor to any dish. You can use any type of cabbage you want, but green cabbage is versatile and can complement any dish without overpowering it.

SERVES 4

Per Serving:

Calories	276
Fat	16g
Sodium	1,051mg
Carbohydrates	3g
Fiber	1g
Sugar	1g
Protein	30g

FOR CABBAGE

- 2 cups chopped green cabbage
- 1 tablespoon extra-virgin olive oil
- 1 teaspoon onion powder
- 1 teaspoon garlic powder
- 1 teaspoon Italian seasoning
- 1 teaspoon sea salt
- ½ teaspoon ground black pepper
- ½ teaspoon red pepper flakes

FOR SALMON

- 4 (4-ounce) salmon fillets, skin removed
- 1 tablespoon extra-virgin olive oil
- 1 teaspoon Italian seasoning
- ½ teaspoon lemon pepper seasoning
- ¼ teaspoon red pepper flakes
- 1 teaspoon sea salt
- ½ teaspoon ground black pepper

1. Preheat oven to 450°F. Line a baking sheet with parchment paper.
2. To make Cabbage: Spread cabbage out on prepared baking sheet, drizzle with oil, and sprinkle with spices. Roast 15 minutes or until cabbage starts to get tender and slightly browned, tossing once halfway during cooking.
3. To make Salmon: Place salmon on top of Cabbage on baking sheet. Drizzle with oil and sprinkle with spices. Bake 12 minutes or until salmon flakes apart easily with a fork. Remove from oven and allow to cool 30 minutes.
4. Transfer equal parts Cabbage and 1 salmon fillet to each of four airtight containers. Cover and store in refrigerator until ready to eat, up to 4 days.
5. When ready to serve, transfer to a skillet, cover, and cook over low heat 5 minutes or until heated through.

Tuna and White Bean Salad

SERVES 4

Per Serving:

Calories	434
Fat	16g
Sodium	822mg
Carbohydrates	34g
Fiber	17g
Sugar	3g
Protein	36g

CILANTRO THE CHELATOR

In addition to adding some pretty serious flavor, cilantro acts as a chelating agent. In other words, compounds in cilantro react to heavy metal ions, turning them into stable water-soluble substances that your body can effectively detoxify. When you combine tuna, which is high in mercury, with cilantro, the cilantro helps negate the effect mercury can have on your body.

Thanks to canned beans and canned tuna, this cold bean salad comes together in minutes with no cooking required. You can eat it as a protein-rich meal on its own or reduce the portion size and pair it with some cooked chicken or steak.

¼ cup extra-virgin olive oil
¼ cup red wine vinegar
1 tablespoon lemon juice
2 cloves garlic, peeled and minced
¼ teaspoon sea salt
¼ teaspoon ground black pepper
2 (5-ounce) cans solid white albacore tuna packed in water, drained
2 (15-ounce) cans cannellini beans, drained and rinsed
2 tablespoons minced red onion
2 tablespoons chopped fresh cilantro
¾ cup halved cherry tomatoes
4 cups fresh arugula

1. Add oil, vinegar, lemon juice, garlic, salt, and pepper to a large mixing bowl. Whisk until smooth. Add tuna, beans, onion, cilantro, and tomatoes. Mix well. Stir in arugula.
2. Divide evenly into four airtight containers. Cover and store in refrigerator until ready to eat, up to 4 days. Serve cold.

Shrimp Cakes

To make these cakes, you can cook shrimp yourself and chop it once it cools, or, to save time, you can buy precooked shrimp in a can or from the seafood counter at the grocery store. The size of the shrimp doesn't matter, as long as you have a pound of cooked meat.

1 pound cooked peeled deveined shrimp, finely chopped
¾ cup almond meal
2 large eggs, lightly beaten
1 tablespoon finely chopped red onion
2 tablespoons Worcestershire sauce
1 tablespoon Tessemae's Mayonnaise
1 tablespoon Dijon mustard
1 teaspoon Old Bay Seasoning
½ teaspoon garlic powder

1. Preheat air fryer to 375°F.
2. Combine all ingredients in a large bowl. Divide into eight equal portions and shape each portion into a patty.
3. Spray air fryer basked with avocado oil cooking spray. Transfer cakes to basket and cook four at a time in air fryer 5 minutes on each side or until golden brown and crispy. Remove from air fryer and allow to cool 30 minutes.
4. Transfer two cakes to each of four separate airtight containers. Cover and store in refrigerator until ready to eat, up to 4 days.
5. When ready to serve, eat cold or return to air fryer basket and cook at 300°F 3 minutes or until heated through.

SERVES 4

Per Serving (2 cakes):

Calories	243
Fat	10g
Sodium	756mg
Carbohydrates	4g
Fiber	0g
Sugar	2g
Protein	33g

SELENIUM IN SHRIMP

A 4-ounce serving of shrimp also contains 54 micrograms of selenium—just 1 microgram short of the entire amount you need for the whole day. Selenium has a number of health benefits—it can reduce your risk of cancer, heart disease, and mental decline—but one of the most notable is its role in thyroid health. Many people with thyroid diseases are deficient in selenium, and research shows that eating enough of the mineral daily can help keep your thyroid functioning properly.

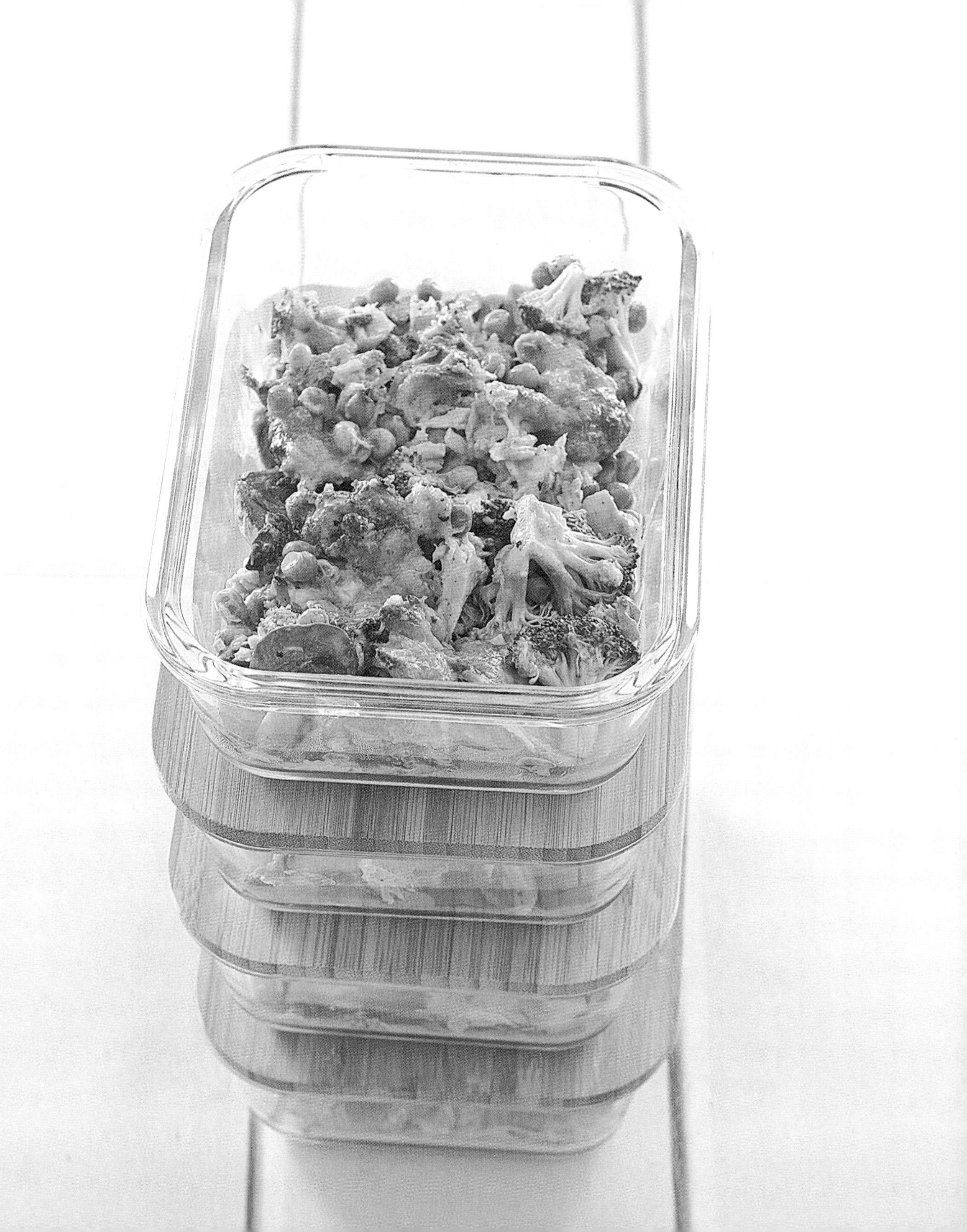

Tuna Broccoli Bake

If you want to switch things up in this recipe, you can replace the tuna with canned salmon (or leftover cooked salmon). The fat macros may go up slightly, but the extra omega-3s are worth it.

SERVES 6

Per Serving:

Calories	351
Fat	26g
Sodium	618mg
Carbohydrates	8g
Fiber	3g
Sugar	3g
Protein	21g

2 (5-ounce) cans solid white albacore tuna packed in water, drained

6 cups broccoli florets

1 cup sliced white mushrooms

1 cup shredded Cheddar cheese, divided

1 cup frozen peas

¾ cup Tessemae's Creamy Ranch Dressing

½ teaspoon sea salt

¼ teaspoon ground black pepper

1. Preheat oven to 375°F.
2. Combine tuna, broccoli, mushrooms, ½ cup cheese, peas, ranch dressing, salt, and pepper in a large bowl and mix well. Transfer to a 9" × 9" baking dish. Sprinkle remaining ½ cup cheese on top.
3. Bake 30 minutes or until casserole is bubbly and cheese is melted. Remove from oven and allow to cool 1 hour.
4. Divide evenly into six airtight containers. Cover and store in refrigerator until ready to eat, up to 4 days.
5. When ready to serve, transfer to a skillet, cover, and cook over low heat 5 minutes or until heated through.

Garlic and Basil Cod

SERVES 4

Per Serving:

Calories	168
Fat	8g
Sodium	441mg
Carbohydrates	3g
Fiber	1g
Sugar	2g
Protein	22g

For the best flavor, you will want to marinate this Garlic and Basil Cod for 1 hour in the refrigerator, so plan accordingly for your cooking day.

4 (4-ounce) boneless cod fillets, skin removed
2 tablespoons extra-virgin olive oil
1 tablespoon lemon juice
1½ teaspoons Old Bay Seasoning
1 teaspoon dried basil
6 cloves garlic, peeled and minced
1 large zucchini, diced
1 large summer squash, diced
½ teaspoon sea salt
¼ teaspoon ground black pepper

1. Put cod in a large zip-top bag. Add oil, lemon juice, Old Bay, basil, and garlic. Massage to combine and coat fish. Seal bag and refrigerate 1 hour.
2. Preheat oven to 425°F. Line a baking sheet with parchment paper.
3. Arrange zucchini and squash on prepared baking sheet in a single layer, leaving room in middle for cod. Spray vegetables with avocado oil cooking spray and sprinkle salt and pepper on top.
4. Place cod in center of sheet and pour marinade on top.
5. Bake 15 minutes or until fish flakes apart easily with a fork. Remove from oven and allow to cool 20 minutes.
6. Divide zucchini and squash evenly into each of four airtight containers. Top each with 1 cod fillet. Cover and store in refrigerator until ready to eat, up to 4 days.
7. When ready to serve, transfer to a skillet, cover, and cook over low heat 5 minutes or until heated through.

Sheet Pan Tilapia and Vegetables

Tilapia is one of the leanest fish, with only 137 calories and 2.4 grams of fat per 4-ounce serving. Each serving still packs 28.6 grams of protein, though, so whenever you need a boost of protein without a bunch of other macros, tilapia is the choice.

SERVES 4

Per Serving:

Calories	211
Fat	11g
Sodium	531mg
Carbohydrates	7g
Fiber	3g
Sugar	4g
Protein	21g

1 pound asparagus, ends trimmed

2 cups cherry tomatoes

4 (4-ounce) tilapia fillets

3 tablespoons unsalted grass-fed butter, melted

2 tablespoons lemon juice

2 teaspoons Italian seasoning

½ teaspoon sea salt

¼ teaspoon ground black pepper

1. Preheat oven to 400°F. Line a baking sheet with parchment paper.
2. Arrange asparagus and tomatoes in a single layer on baking sheet. Place tilapia on top.
3. Whisk together remaining ingredients in a small bowl, then pour over vegetables and fish.
4. Roast 15 minutes or until tilapia flakes apart easily with a fork and asparagus is tender. Remove from oven and allow to cool 20 minutes.
5. Transfer equal portions of vegetables to each of four airtight containers. Top each with 1 tilapia fillet. Cover and store in refrigerator until ready to eat, up to 4 days.
6. When ready to serve, transfer to a skillet, cover, and cook over low heat 5 minutes or until heated through.

Quinoa and Tuna Casserole

SERVES 4

Per Serving:

Calories	480
Fat	11g
Sodium	903mg
Carbohydrates	56g
Fiber	8g
Sugar	10g
Protein	39g

Unlike other casseroles that rely on canned creamed soups, this Quinoa and Tuna Casserole is made with a quick, macro-friendly homemade broth that comes together in minutes. And since the quinoa goes into the oven uncooked, there isn't a lot of prep time involved.

1 cup uncooked sprouted quinoa, rinsed

1 pound bite-sized broccoli florets

2 (5-ounce) cans solid white albacore tuna packed in water, drained

3⁄4 cup frozen peas

1 cup chicken broth

2 tablespoons arrowroot powder

1½ cups organic 1% milk

1 teaspoon garlic powder

1 teaspoon sea salt

½ teaspoon ground black pepper

½ teaspoon chili powder

½ cup shredded Cheddar cheese

1. Preheat oven to 350°F. Spray a 9" × 13" baking dish with avocado oil cooking spray.
2. Pour quinoa into baking dish and spread out evenly. Top with broccoli and tuna. Sprinkle peas on top. Set aside.
3. Heat broth in a small saucepan over medium heat 3 minutes. Add arrowroot and whisk until smooth. Continue whisking and cooking another 4 minutes or until broth starts to thicken. Whisk in milk, garlic powder, salt, pepper, and chili powder. Reduce heat to low and cook 3 minutes, stirring frequently. Pour sauce over tuna. Sprinkle cheese on top.
4. Bake 40 minutes or until casserole is hot and bubbly and quinoa is fluffy. Remove from oven and allow to cool 1 hour.
5. Divide evenly into four airtight containers. Cover and store in refrigerator until ready to eat, up to 4 days.
6. When ready to serve, transfer to a skillet, cover, and cook over medium-low heat 5 minutes or until heated through.

MORE ON MERCURY

Mercury in more than trace amounts is harmful because it binds to selenium and prevents the mineral from performing its duties in your brain (negatively affecting motor performance, cognition, memory, and coordination). If you eat fish with a high selenium-to-mercury ratio (meaning it contains more selenium than mercury), the harmful effect is partly negated. Most fish, contain more selenium than mercury. Albacore, skipjack, and yellowfin tuna have the highest selenium-to-mercury ratio. Shark, tilefish, king mackerel, and swordfish have the lowest ratio.

Mustard-Crusted Salmon with Roasted Asparagus

SERVES 4

Per Serving:

Calories	247
Fat	10g
Sodium	518mg
Carbohydrates	7g
Fiber	4g
Sugar	2g
Protein	32g

Asparagus is one of the highest-protein green vegetables you can eat, with 1 cup of chopped spears containing 4.26 grams. Because of that, this combo meal of salmon and asparagus is a great source of protein and healthy fats.

FOR ASPARAGUS

1 teaspoon extra-virgin olive oil

2 cloves garlic, peeled and minced

1 pound asparagus, ends trimmed

¼ teaspoon red pepper flakes

FOR SALMON

4 (4-ounce) salmon fillets, skin removed

2 tablespoons Dijon mustard

1 teaspoon ChocZero Maple-Flavored Syrup

½ teaspoon sea salt

¼ teaspoon ground black pepper

¼ teaspoon paprika

1. To make Asparagus: Preheat oven to 350°F. Line a baking sheet with parchment paper.
2. Combine oil and garlic in a large bowl. Add asparagus and toss to coat. Sprinkle red pepper flakes on top and mix well.
3. Arrange asparagus on prepared baking sheet in a single layer. Bake 5 minutes.
4. To make Salmon: Push asparagus to sides of sheet and arrange salmon in center.
5. Combine mustard and maple syrup in a small bowl and brush on salmon. Sprinkle salmon with salt, black pepper, and paprika.
6. Bake 15 minutes or until salmon flakes apart easily with a fork and asparagus is tender. Remove from oven and allow to cool 20 minutes.
7. Divide asparagus into four airtight containers. Place 1 salmon fillet on top of each. Cover and store in refrigerator until ready to eat, up to 4 days.
8. When ready to serve, transfer to a skillet, cover, and cook over low heat 5 minutes or until heated through.

Blood Orange Baked Salmon

SERVES 4

Per Serving:

Calories	267
Fat	15g
Sodium	621mg
Carbohydrates	4g
Fiber	0g
Sugar	2g
Protein	29g

If you can't find blood oranges, you can use navel oranges in this recipe. Try to freshly squeeze your own orange juice rather than buying it bottled, though. It will make a welcome difference in the taste.

4 (4-ounce) salmon fillets, skin removed
1 teaspoon sea salt
½ teaspoon ground black pepper
4 slices medium blood orange
2 tablespoons unsalted grass-fed butter
1 small shallot, peeled and minced
2 teaspoons minced fresh rosemary
½ cup freshly squeezed blood orange juice
1 tablespoon lemon juice
1 tablespoon coconut aminos
1 teaspoon rice vinegar
2 cloves garlic, peeled and minced
½ teaspoon grated fresh ginger

1. Preheat oven to 400°F. Line a baking sheet with parchment paper.
2. Arrange salmon on prepared baking sheet and sprinkle with salt and pepper. Put 1 slice blood orange on top of each fillet. Bake 15 minutes or until salmon flakes apart easily with a fork. Allow salmon to cool slightly, about 15 minutes.
3. While salmon is cooking, melt butter in a medium skillet over medium heat. Add shallot and rosemary and cook 2 minutes. Add remaining ingredients and bring to a boil. Reduce heat to low and simmer until sauce thickens, about 5 minutes. Allow to cool 10 minutes.
4. Transfer 1 salmon fillet to each of four airtight containers. Pour equal amounts of sauce on top. Cover and store in refrigerator until ready to eat, up to 4 days.
5. When ready to serve, transfer to a skillet, cover, and cook over low heat 5 minutes or until heated through.

THE BENEFITS OF BLOOD ORANGES

Blood oranges are natural mutations of sweet oranges. They have a crimson-colored inner flesh, hence the name. The color comes from extra anthocyanins, a family of polyphenols that typically aren't found in citrus fruits. Anthocyanins have been shown to help reduce your risk of heart disease, balance blood sugar, promote weight loss, stave off inflammation, and prevent cancer.

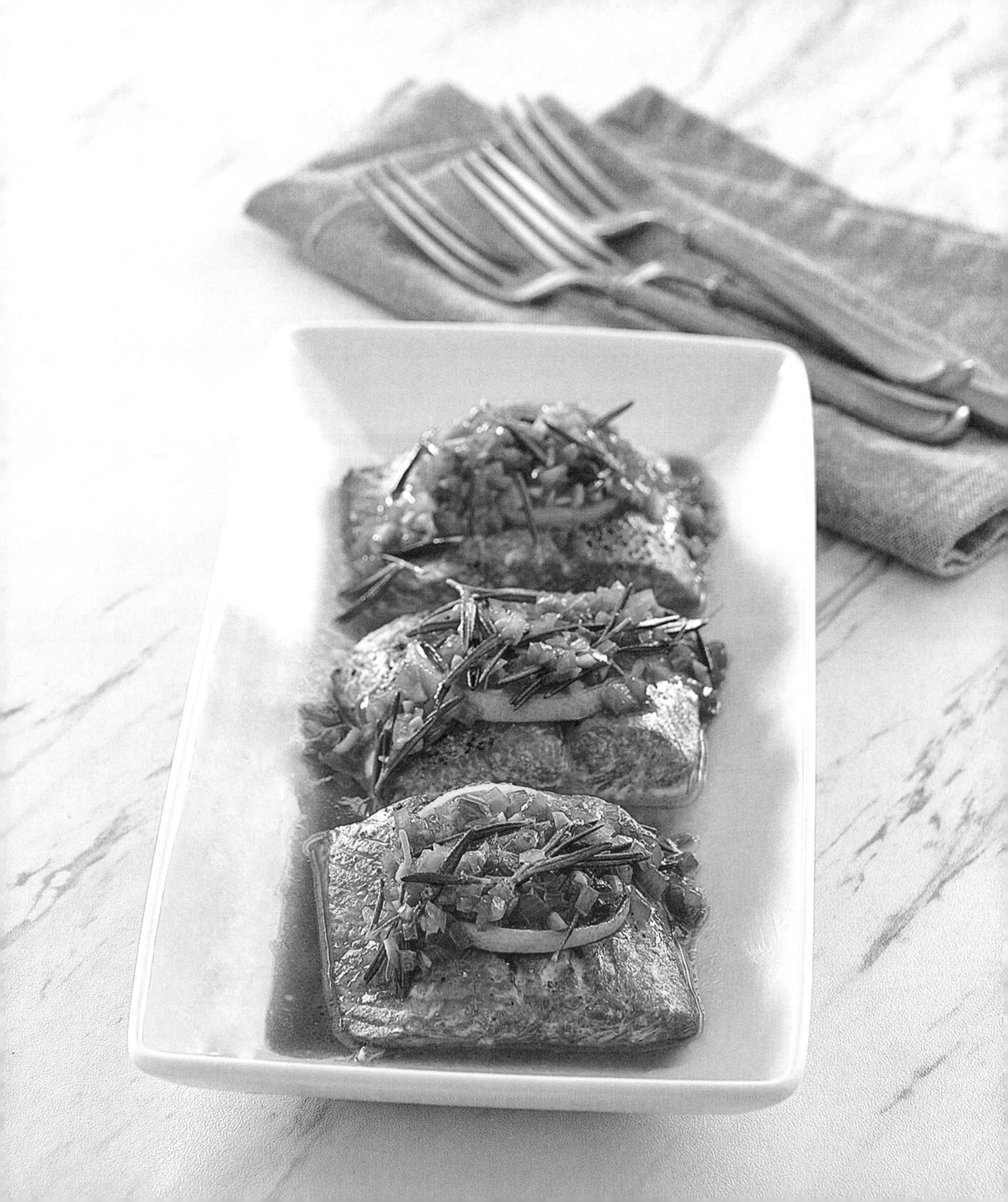

Mediterranean Salmon with Quinoa

SERVES 4

Per Serving:

Calories	564
Fat	29g
Sodium	491mg
Carbohydrates	40g
Fiber	3g
Sugar	6g
Protein	36g

If you want to cut back on carbs a bit, you can serve this salmon with cauliflower rice instead of quinoa. On the flip side, swapping out the quinoa for regular rice will up the carbs slightly, by about 6 grams per cup.

FOR SALMON

4 (4-ounce) salmon fillets, skins removed

¼ cup extra-virgin olive oil

2 tablespoons balsamic vinegar

4 cloves garlic, peeled and minced

2 tablespoons chopped fresh basil

¼ cup diced Roma tomatoes

1 teaspoon garlic powder

½ teaspoon sea salt

FOR QUINOA

2 cups chicken broth

1 cup sprouted quinoa, rinsed

2 tablespoons minced green onion

⅓ cup crumbled feta cheese

1. To make Salmon: Preheat broiler to low.
2. Arrange salmon in a single layer in a 9" × 13" baking dish. Whisk together oil, vinegar, and garlic in a small bowl. Pour over salmon.
3. Combine basil, tomatoes, garlic powder, and salt in a medium bowl. Scoop tomato mixture on top of salmon.
4. Broil 15 minutes or until salmon flakes apart easily with a fork.
5. To make Quinoa: While salmon is cooking, pour broth into a small saucepan. Bring to a boil over medium-high heat. Stir in quinoa, reduce heat to low, cover, and cook 10 minutes. Remove from heat and let sit, covered, 5 minutes.
6. Fluff quinoa with a fork and divide evenly into each of four airtight containers. Top each with 1 salmon fillet. Sprinkle green onion and feta over each salmon fillet. Cover and store in refrigerator until ready to eat, up to 4 days.
7. When ready to serve, transfer to a skillet, cover, and cook over low heat 5 minutes or until heated through.

Easy Tuna Patties

Thanks to the air fryer and a handful of easy-to-grab ingredients, these tuna patties couldn't be easier to make. They take only about 10 minutes to whip up and will feed you for days. Throw them on salads or serve between a couple slices of your favorite macro-friendly bread.

SERVES 4

Per Serving (2 patties):

Calories	109
Fat	5g
Sodium	616mg
Carbohydrates	1g
Fiber	0g
Sugar	0g
Protein	15g

2 (5-ounce) cans solid white albacore tuna packed in water, drained

2 tablespoons minced yellow onion

2 large eggs, lightly beaten

2 tablespoons yellow mustard

⅓ cup almond meal

1 teaspoon sea salt

½ teaspoon ground black pepper

¼ teaspoon paprika

1. Preheat air fryer to 400°F.
2. Combine all ingredients in a large bowl. Divide mixture into eight equal portions and shape into patties.
3. Spray air fryer basket with avocado oil cooking spray and cook patties, four at a time, 3 minutes on each side or until golden brown and crispy. Remove from air fryer and allow to cool 20 minutes.
4. Transfer two patties to each of four airtight containers. Cover and store in refrigerator until ready to eat, up to 4 days.
5. When ready to serve, cook 3 minutes in air fryer at 300°F or until heated through.

Garlic Butter Salmon and Vegetables

SERVES 6

Per Serving:

Calories	313
Fat	17g
Sodium	897mg
Carbohydrates	8g
Fiber	3g
Sugar	4g
Protein	31g

This recipe yields six meals in about 45 minutes. Double up for the week by making one dish with salmon and another with chicken.

FOR VEGETABLES

1 pound asparagus, ends trimmed

2 cups cauliflower florets

4 medium carrots, peeled and cut into coins

2 teaspoons extra-virgin olive oil

1 teaspoon sea salt

½ teaspoon ground black pepper

FOR SALMON

3 tablespoons unsalted grass-fed butter, melted

5 cloves garlic, peeled and minced

1 tablespoon fresh lemon juice

1 teaspoon dried rosemary

½ teaspoon dried parsley

1 teaspoon sea salt

½ teaspoon ground black pepper

6 (4-ounce) salmon fillets, skin removed

6 lemon slices

1. To make Vegetables: Preheat oven to 400°F. Line a baking sheet with parchment paper.
2. Combine asparagus, cauliflower, and carrots in a large bowl. Drizzle with oil and sprinkle salt and pepper on top. Toss to coat evenly.
3. Spread vegetables out in a single layer on prepared baking sheet. Bake 15 minutes.
4. To make Salmon: While vegetables are cooking, whisk together butter, garlic, lemon juice, rosemary, parsley, salt, and pepper in a small bowl.
5. Push vegetables to sides of sheet and arrange salmon in center. Pour butter mixture on top of salmon and place 1 lemon slice on top of each fillet.
6. Bake 15 minutes or until salmon flakes apart easily with a fork. Remove from oven and allow to cool 20 minutes.
7. Scoop equal amounts of vegetables into each of six airtight containers. Top each with 1 salmon fillet. Cover and store in refrigerator until ready to eat, up to 1 week.
8. When ready to serve, transfer to a skillet, cover, and cook over low heat 5 minutes or until heated through.

Sweet Chili Salmon

This salmon requires a couple hours of marinating time, so make sure you account for this preparation when you're planning your cooking day.

SERVES 4

Per Serving:

Calories	225
Fat	10g
Sodium	533mg
Carbohydrates	4g
Fiber	0g
Sugar	2g
Protein	30g

4 (4-ounce) salmon fillets, skin removed
½ teaspoon sea salt
¼ teaspoon ground black pepper
⅓ cup Yai's Thai Sweet Chili Sauce
2 tablespoons coconut aminos
2 cloves garlic, peeled and minced
2 tablespoons chopped scallions

1. Arrange salmon in an ungreased 9" × 9" baking dish. Sprinkle with salt and pepper.
2. Combine chili sauce, coconut aminos, garlic, and scallions in a small bowl, then pour over salmon. Cover and refrigerate 2 hours.
3. Preheat oven broiler to low. Line a baking sheet with parchment paper.
4. Remove salmon from marinade (discard marinade) and transfer to prepared baking sheet. Broil 7 minutes or until fish flakes apart easily with a fork. Remove from oven and allow to cool 20 minutes.
5. Transfer 1 salmon fillet to each of four airtight containers. Cover and store in refrigerator until ready to eat, up to 4 days.
6. When ready to serve, transfer to a skillet, cover, and cook over low heat 5 minutes or until heated through.

Garlic Herb Yogurt Cod

SERVES 4

Per Serving:

Calories	146
Fat	9g
Sodium	894mg
Carbohydrates	1g
Fiber	0g
Sugar	1g
Protein	15g

When you're making this cod, you can roast a big sheet of your favorite vegetables—whatever you have in the refrigerator—and have dinner for the week ready in less than 30 minutes. If you have room for some carbs, add rice or potatoes.

4 (4-ounce) cod fillets

1 teaspoon sea salt

½ teaspoon ground black pepper

3 tablespoons 1% plain Greek yogurt

2 tablespoons unsalted grass-fed butter, melted

2 tablespoons lemon juice

1 tablespoon grated Parmesan cheese

4 cloves garlic, peeled and minced

1 teaspoon dried basil

¼ teaspoon Italian seasoning

⅛ teaspoon red pepper flakes

1. Preheat oven to 400°F. Spray a 9" × 13" baking dish with avocado oil cooking spray.
2. Arrange cod in a single layer in baking dish. Sprinkle with salt and pepper.
3. Whisk remaining ingredients in a medium bowl until smooth. Spoon over fillets.
4. Bake 10 minutes or until cod flakes apart easily with a fork. Remove from oven and allow to cool 20 minutes.
5. Transfer 1 fillet to each of four airtight containers. Spoon butter mixture over fillets, cover, and store in refrigerator until ready to eat, up to 1 week.
6. When ready to serve, transfer to a skillet, cover, and cook over low heat 5 minutes or until heated through.

Baked Teriyaki Salmon

Salmon is one of the fattiest fish you can eat, but most of that fat is in the form of omega-3 fatty acids, which are vital for your brain. But if you can't fit the extra fat into your macros, you can swap in a lower-fat white fish.

SERVES 4

Per Serving:

Calories	318
Fat	17g
Sodium	224mg
Carbohydrates	16g
Fiber	14g
Sugar	3g
Protein	25g

4 (4-ounce) boneless salmon fillets, skin removed
¼ cup ChocZero Maple-Flavored Syrup
3 tablespoons coconut aminos
1 tablespoon extra-virgin olive oil
1 teaspoon Worcestershire sauce
2 teaspoons minced fresh ginger
½ teaspoon ground black pepper

1. Preheat oven to 375°F. Line a 9" × 9" baking dish with parchment paper, leaving extra hanging over the edges.
2. Arrange salmon in a single layer in prepared baking dish.
3. Fold up parchment paper to cover fillets. Crimp edges to seal. Bake 15 minutes. Remove baking dish from oven and turn oven to low broil.
4. Whisk together remaining ingredients in a small bowl. Open parchment paper and spoon sauce over salmon. Broil 3 minutes. Remove from oven and allow to cool 20 minutes.
5. Transfer 1 salmon fillet to each of four airtight containers. Cover and store in refrigerator until ready to eat, up to 4 days.
6. When ready to serve, transfer to a skillet, cover, and cook over low heat 5 minutes or until heated through.

THE POWER OF OMEGA-3S

Omega-3s are considered essential fatty acids because you have to get them from food or supplements since your body doesn't make them. Along with keeping your brain healthy, omega-3 fatty acids have been shown to reduce the risk of heart disease, improve insulin resistance, fight inflammation, help control blood sugar, improve anxiety and depression, and contribute to healthy joints. Other foods that are high in omega-3s are mackerel, herring, oysters, sardines, anchovies, flaxseeds, chia seeds, and walnuts.

CHAPTER 8

Vegetarian and Vegan Main Meals

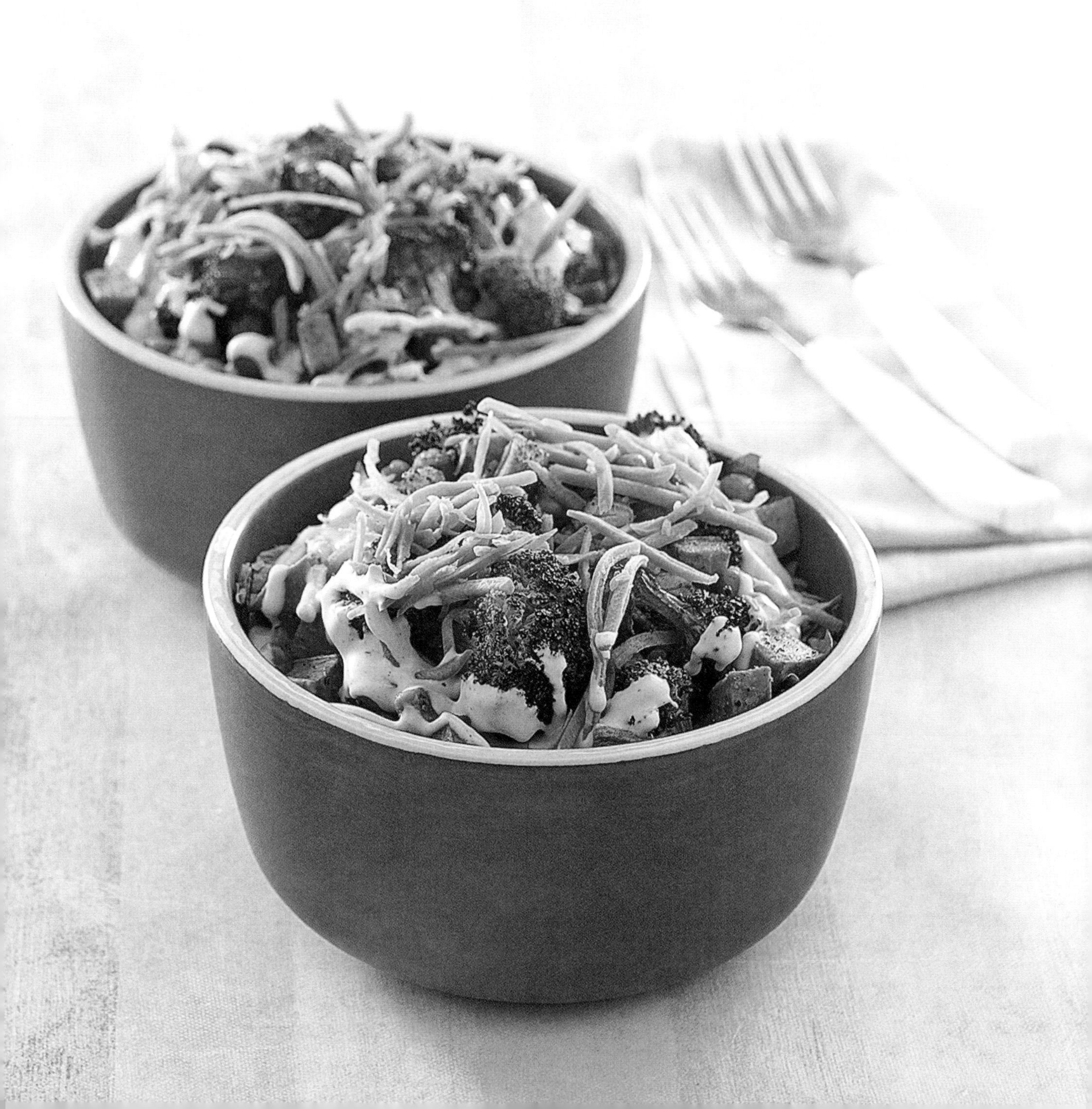

Broccoli Chickpea Pesto Bowls

If you want some additional protein, you can also add your favorite tofu to these bowls. And any ranch dressing will work as a drizzle, but the Habanero Ranch gives it a nice little kick.

SERVES 6

Per Serving:

Calories	423
Fat	20g
Sodium	826mg
Carbohydrates	53g
Fiber	10g
Sugar	7g
Protein	7g

2 large sweet potatoes, peeled and cubed
1 large yellow onion, peeled and diced
3 cups bite-sized broccoli florets
3 cloves garlic, peeled and minced
1 (15-ounce) can chickpeas, drained and rinsed
2 teaspoons avocado oil
1 teaspoon chili powder
1 teaspoon sea salt
½ teaspoon ground black pepper
½ teaspoon garlic powder
3 cups cooked sprouted brown rice
3 cups chopped fresh spinach
¾ cup peeled shredded carrots
¾ cup Tessemae's Habanero Ranch dressing

1. Preheat oven to 400°F. Line a baking sheet with parchment paper.
2. Combine sweet potatoes, onion, broccoli, garlic, and chickpeas in a large bowl. Drizzle with oil and toss to coat. Spread out evenly on prepared baking sheet. Sprinkle with chili powder, salt, pepper, and garlic powder.
3. Bake 25 minutes or until broccoli is tender and chickpeas are roasted. Remove from oven and allow to cool 20 minutes.
4. Scoop ½ cup brown rice and ½ cup chopped spinach into each of six airtight containers. Top with equal parts roasted vegetable mixture and 2 tablespoons carrots.
5. Pour 2 tablespoons dressing into each of six small containers. Place small containers in large containers, cover, and store in refrigerator until ready to eat, up to 1 week.
6. When ready to serve, drizzle dressing on top of bowl.

Chickpea Quinoa Salad

SERVES 6

Per Serving:

Calories	409
Fat	13g
Sodium	295mg
Carbohydrates	53g
Fiber	15g
Sugar	5g
Protein	20g

The homemade dressing gives this Chickpea Quinoa Salad a nice flavor and adds some extra protein, thanks to the almond butter, but if you want to save some time or you don't have some of the ingredients on hand, you can use any of your favorite dressings that fit into your plan.

FOR DRESSING

⅓ cup light coconut milk

3 tablespoons no-sugar-added almond butter

2 tablespoons coconut aminos

2 tablespoons lime juice

1 tablespoon red curry paste

1 teaspoon toasted sesame oil

½ teaspoon ground cumin

FOR BOWLS

3 cups cooked sprouted quinoa

2 (15-ounce) cans chickpeas, drained and rinsed

1½ cups peeled shredded carrots

6 tablespoons hemp seeds

6 cups mixed greens

1. To make Dressing: Whisk all ingredients in a medium bowl until smooth. Divide evenly into six quart-sized Mason jars.
2. To make Bowls: Scoop ½ cup quinoa, ½ cup chickpeas, ¼ cup carrots, and 1 tablespoon hemp seeds into each jar. Top each with 1 cup mixed greens. Cover and store in refrigerator until ready to eat, up to 1 week.
3. When ready to serve, shake vigorously to combine ingredients and coat with Dressing.

A RARE COMPLETE PROTEIN

Hemp is one of the rare plant proteins that's a complete protein, meaning it contains all nine of the essential amino acids. While hemp provides a hefty dose of protein, it's also fairly high in fat—2 tablespoons has 14.6 grams of fat and 9.5 grams of protein. Don't let that deter you from eating it, though. If you don't eat meat and you're trying to get enough high-quality protein, hemp is one of your best bets.

Cajun Mac and Cheese

This recipe makes more Cajun Mac and Cheese than you might be able to eat in a week. Portion everything out and then freeze what you won't eat within a week.

SERVES 12

Per Serving:

Calories	132
Fat	5g
Sodium	386mg
Carbohydrates	13g
Fiber	2g
Sugar	2g
Protein	9g

8 ounces Banza pasta shells

1 tablespoon unsalted grass-fed butter

2 teaspoons gluten-free flour

½ cup organic 1% milk

¾ cup shredded pepper Jack cheese

2 teaspoons Slap Ya Mama Cajun Seasoning

2 teaspoons paprika

½ teaspoon sea salt

½ teaspoon ground black pepper

1 cup 2% plain Greek yogurt

2 tablespoons cream cheese, softened

2 teaspoons mustard powder

½ cup chopped roasted red peppers

1. Preheat oven to 400°F. Spray a 9" × 9" baking dish with avocado oil cooking spray. Set aside.
2. Bring a large pot of water to a boil over high heat. Reduce heat to medium-high and add pasta. Cook 5 minutes, drain, and transfer to prepared baking dish.
3. Melt butter in a medium skillet over medium-high heat. Add flour and cook 2 minutes, whisking constantly. Pour in milk and reduce heat to medium-low. Cook, whisking constantly, 7 minutes or until mixture starts to thicken.
4. Add half of cheese to skillet and stir until smooth. Add remaining cheese and keep stirring until smooth. Stir in Cajun seasoning, paprika, salt, and pepper until smooth. Add remaining ingredients and cook until cream cheese melts, about 3 minutes.
5. Pour sauce mixture over pasta and toss to coat evenly. Bake 20 minutes or until sauce is bubbly and top starts to turn golden brown. Remove from oven and allow to cool 30 minutes.
6. Divide mixture into twelve airtight containers. Cover and store in refrigerator up to 1 week, or in freezer up to 3 months.
7. When ready to serve, transfer to a saucepan, cover, and cook over low heat 5 minutes or until heated through.

Eggplant Casserole

SERVES 6

Per Serving:

Calories	143
Fat	6g
Sodium	651mg
Carbohydrates	15g
Fiber	7g
Sugar	9g
Protein	7g

SMALL VERSUS LARGE EGGPLANTS

A large eggplant may seem like a logical substitution for two small ones, but the size makes a difference in taste and texture. Larger eggplants are less flavorful and have tougher skin—it's still edible but not as pleasant to eat. If you do use a large eggplant, you may want to peel it before adding it to your recipes. When picking out an eggplant, feel it and make sure it's a little firm, but not too hard.

Rather than layering eggplant in a lasagna-like fashion, this vegetarian casserole highlights the rich flavor of the vegetable.

- 2 small eggplants
- 2 teaspoons extra-virgin olive oil
- 2 large shallots, peeled and minced
- 4 cloves garlic, peeled and minced
- 1 small jalapeño, seeded and minced
- 1 medium stalk celery, finely chopped
- ¼ cup dry white wine
- 1 (15-ounce) can petite-diced tomatoes, drained
- 3 tablespoons tomato paste
- 1 tablespoon Italian seasoning
- 1 teaspoon sea salt
- ½ teaspoon ground black pepper
- 2 cups chopped fresh spinach
- 1 (15-ounce) can cannellini beans, drained and rinsed
- ½ cup shredded mozzarella cheese

1. Preheat oven to 400°F.
2. Place eggplants in a 9" × 13" baking dish and roast 45 minutes or until tender. Remove from oven and allow to cool slightly, about 10 minutes. Cut off stem end of eggplant and then roughly chop, leaving skin on.
3. Heat oil in a large saucepan over medium heat. Add shallots, garlic, jalapeño, and celery and cook until celery starts to soften, about 4 minutes. Stir in wine and cook another 2 minutes.
4. Add chopped eggplant, tomatoes, tomato paste, Italian seasoning, salt, and pepper. Cook 2 minutes. Use an immersion blender to lightly blend. Make sure not to purée it; just do a few quick pulses to break down the eggplant a bit.
5. Stir in spinach and beans and transfer to a 9" × 13" casserole dish. Sprinkle cheese on top.
6. Bake 25 minutes or until casserole is bubbly and cheese starts to turn golden brown. Remove from oven and allow to cool 1 hour.
7. Divide evenly into each of six airtight containers. Cover and store in refrigerator until ready to eat, up to 1 week.
8. When ready to serve, transfer to a skillet, cover, and cook over low heat 5 minutes or until heated through.

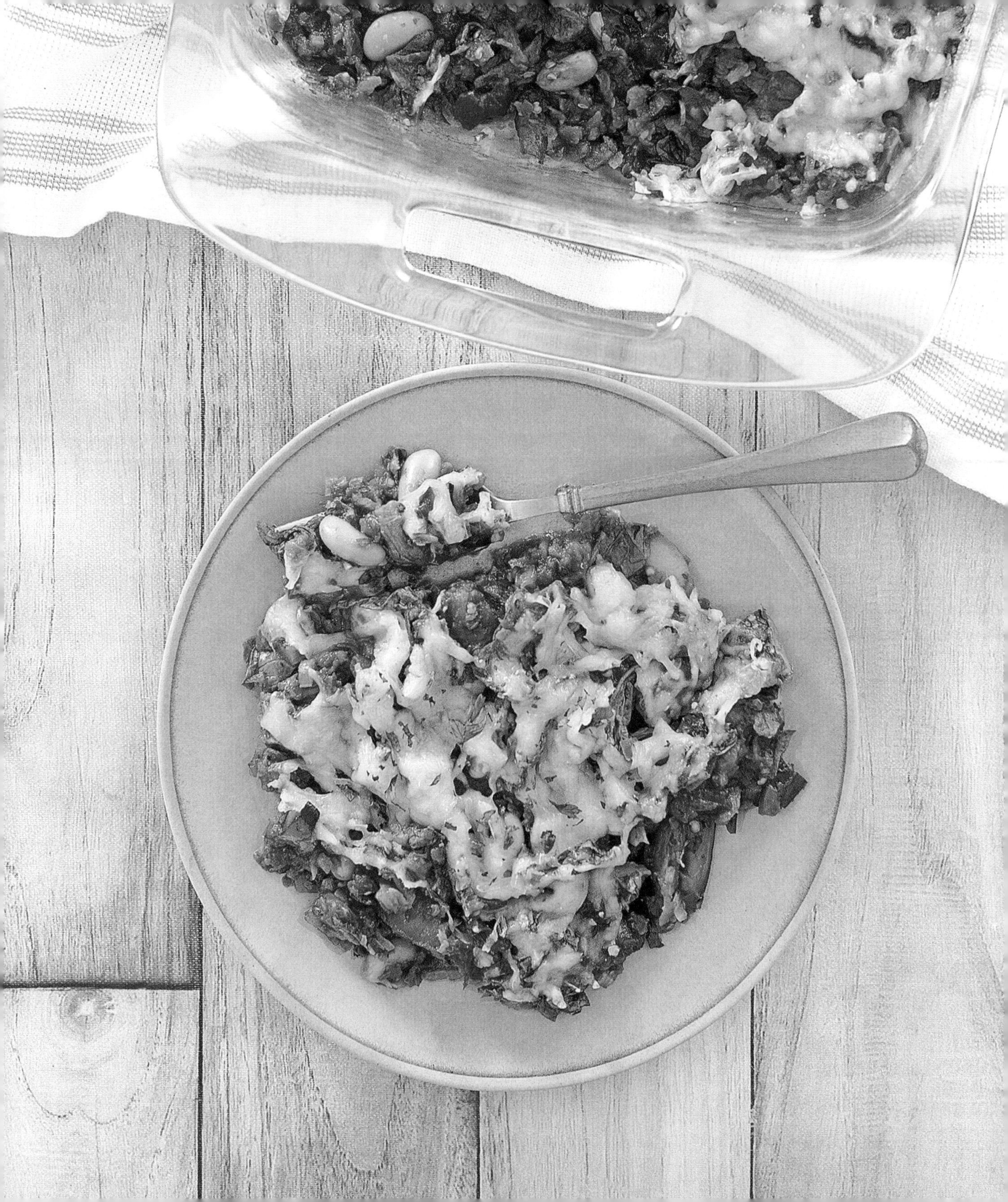

Greek Lentil Salad

SERVES 6

Per Serving:

Calories	425
Fat	25g
Sodium	403mg
Carbohydrates	28g
Fiber	15g
Sugar	2g
Protein	22g

THE DIFFERENT COLORS OF LENTILS

There are four main categories/colors of lentils: brown, green, red, and yellow. Brown and green lentils stand up to cooking and hold their shape better than red and yellow varieties. If cooked too long, red and yellow lentils turn into mush, so they're best in soups, stews, or any dishes where they'll be puréed.

If you want to add some extra protein to this salad, you can throw in ½ cup of chickpeas on top of the lentils. For some crunch, add a handful of nuts or sunflower seeds.

¾ cup Primal Kitchen Greek Vinaigrette and Marinade
4½ cups cooked brown lentils
1½ cups halved cherry tomatoes
1½ cups diced cucumbers
1½ cups kalamata olives
¾ cup crumbled feta cheese
6 tablespoons minced red onion
6 cups fresh baby spinach

1. Pour 2 tablespoons dressing into each of six quart-sized Mason jars.
2. Top each jar with ¾ cup lentils, ¼ cup tomatoes, ¼ cup cucumber, ¼ cup olives, 2 tablespoons feta, 1 tablespoon red onion, and 1 cup spinach.
3. Cover and store in refrigerator until ready to eat, up to 1 week.
4. When ready to serve, shake vigorously to combine ingredients and coat with dressing.

Protein Pasta with White Sauce

Even though Banza pasta is high in protein, it's also fairly high in carbs. If the carb count of this dish is too high for your macros as is, you can substitute a low-carb pasta substitute, like zucchini noodles or spaghetti squash.

SERVES 4

Per Serving:

Calories	342
Fat	9g
Sodium	860mg
Carbohydrates	39g
Fiber	5g
Sugar	5g
Protein	26g

8 ounces Banza penne
2 cups small-curd cottage cheese
½ cup unsweetened almond milk
⅓ cup shredded Parmesan cheese
3 cloves garlic, peeled and minced
1 teaspoon dried oregano
½ teaspoon sea salt
½ teaspoon ground black pepper
2 cups chopped fresh spinach

1. Bring a medium pot of water to a boil over high heat. Add pasta and cook according to package instructions.
2. While pasta is cooking, add cottage cheese, almond milk, Parmesan, garlic, oregano, salt, and pepper to a food processor. Process until smooth.
3. When pasta is done cooking, drain and return to pot. Pour cheese sauce on top and stir to coat. Stir in spinach. Remove from heat and allow to cool 20 minutes.
4. Divide evenly into four airtight containers. Cover and store in refrigerator up to 1 week, until ready to eat.
5. When ready to serve, transfer to a skillet, cover, and cook over low heat 5 minutes or until heated through.

A PROTEIN POWERHOUSE

Cottage cheese is loaded with protein—1 cup of small-curd cottage cheese has 25 grams, and large-curd isn't far behind with 23 grams per cup. The problem is that cottage cheese isn't well liked by many people. If this includes you, sneak it into sauces and casserole dishes. You'll get the added protein and the extra creaminess, but you'll never even know it's there.

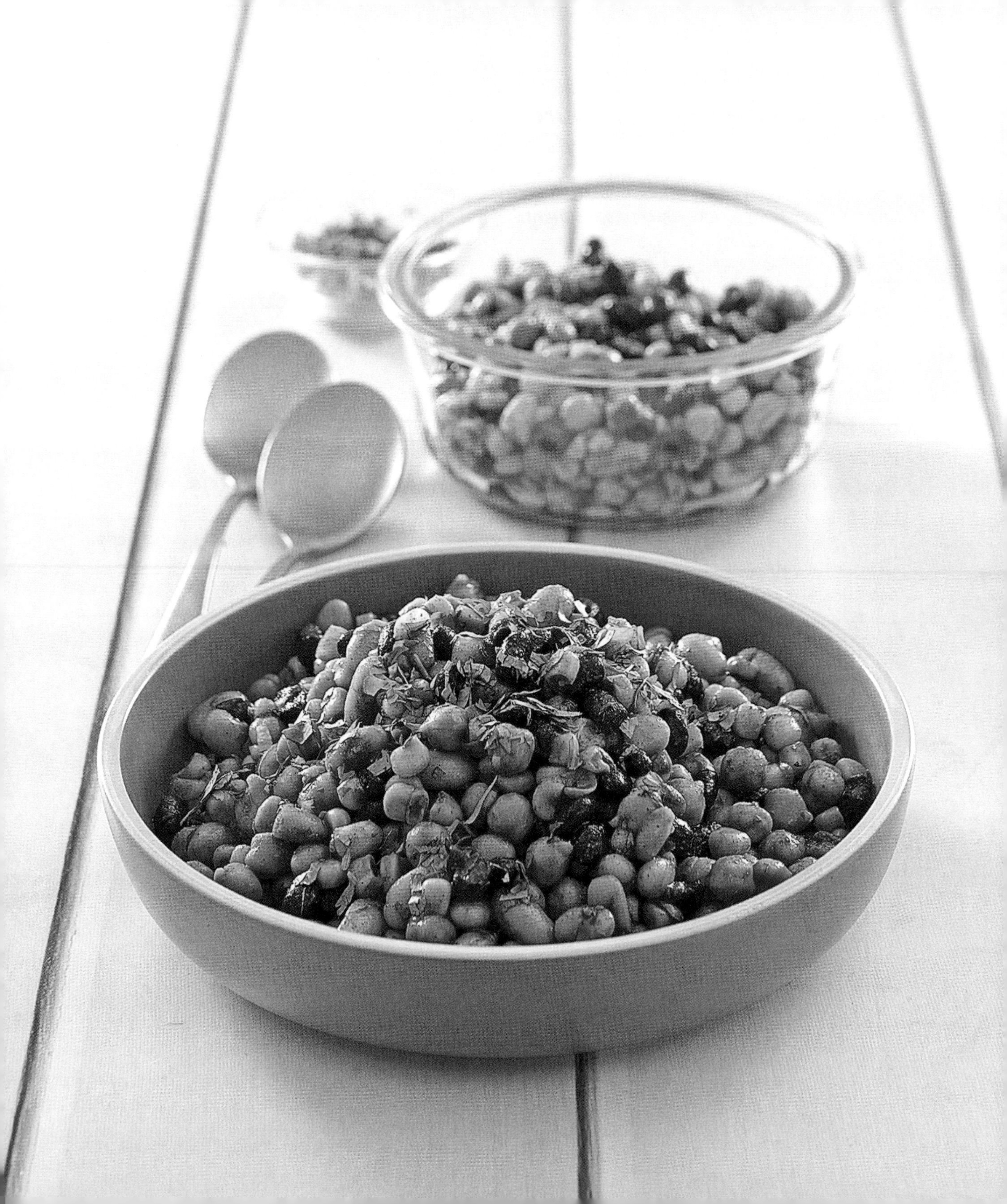

Chili Lime Three-Bean Salad

This Chili Lime Three-Bean Salad comes together in minutes and is so versatile. It has all the macros to be a complete meal on its own, but you can also eat a smaller portion as a side dish for any of your favorite heartier meals. Feel free to add some finely chopped cilantro as a garnish.

SERVES 6

Per Serving:

Calories	230
Fat	3g
Sodium	285mg
Carbohydrates	37g
Fiber	12g
Sugar	2g
Protein	13g

1 (15-ounce) can black beans, drained and rinsed

1 (15-ounce) can cannellini beans, drained and rinsed

1 (15-ounce) can chickpeas, drained and rinsed

1 cup fire-roasted corn kernels

4 cloves garlic, peeled and minced

¼ cup lime juice

1 teaspoon grated lime zest

2 teaspoons extra-virgin olive oil

1 teaspoon ChocZero Maple-Flavored Syrup

1 teaspoon chili powder

½ teaspoon paprika

¼ teaspoon ground cumin

1. Combine black beans, cannellini beans, chickpeas, and corn in a large bowl.
2. In a separate large bowl, whisk together remaining ingredients, then pour over bean mixture. Toss to coat.
3. Divide evenly into six airtight containers. Cover and store in refrigerator until ready to eat, up to 1 week.
4. Serve cold.

Deviled Egg Salad

SERVES 6

Per Serving:

Calories	185
Fat	13g
Sodium	496mg
Carbohydrates	3g
Fiber	0g
Sugar	1g
Protein	14g

If you have some room in your carb allowance, this Deviled Egg Salad goes really well with plantain chips or tostones. You can also wrap it up in a lavash flatbread, serve it with lettuce wraps or on top of a salad, or just eat it as is with a fork.

12 large hard-boiled eggs, peeled and chopped

2 tablespoons Tessemae's Mayonnaise

2 tablespoons 2% plain Greek yogurt

2 tablespoons Dijon mustard

1 tablespoon sweet relish

1 medium scallion, finely chopped

¼ teaspoon Frank's RedHot sauce

½ teaspoon sea salt

¼ teaspoon ground black pepper

1. Combine all ingredients in a large bowl. Divide evenly into six airtight containers.
2. Cover and store in refrigerator until ready to eat, up to 1 week.
3. Serve cold.

Hummus Protein Bowls

SERVES 6

Per Serving:

Calories	317
Fat	12g
Sodium	835mg
Carbohydrates	42g
Fiber	8g
Sugar	1g
Protein	10g

These bowls require almost no cooking, except for the 15 minutes it takes to prep the quinoa. Feel free to add whatever vegetables you have on hand and top it with a Greek or Italian dressing that fits into your macro allowance when you're ready to eat.

3 cups cooked sprouted quinoa

1 (15-ounce) can chickpeas drained and rinsed

1½ cups kalamata olives

¾ cup quartered cucumber slices

¾ cup chopped yellow bell pepper

3 tablespoons chopped red onion

¾ cup garlic hummus

1. Add ½ cup quinoa, ¼ cup chickpeas, ¼ cup olives, 2 tablespoons cucumber, 2 tablespoons bell pepper, 1½ tablespoons red onion, and 2 tablespoons hummus to each of six airtight containers.
2. Cover and store in refrigerator until ready to eat, up to 1 week. Serve cold.

Black Bean and Rice Skillet

This recipe is vegan as written, but you can stir in some cheese right before removing the skillet from the heat if you're vegetarian. If you have some extra fat allowance, add some sliced avocado and/or sliced black olives before serving.

SERVES 6

Per Serving:

Calories	313
Fat	4g
Sodium	747mg
Carbohydrates	59g
Fiber	6g
Sugar	3g
Protein	10g

2 teaspoons avocado oil

3 cloves garlic, peeled and minced

1 small jalapeño, seeded and minced

1 medium yellow onion, finely chopped

1½ cups brown rice

1½ cups vegetable broth

1 (15-ounce) can black beans, drained and rinsed

1 (14.5-ounce) can petite-diced tomatoes

1 teaspoon sea salt

½ teaspoon ground black pepper

1 teaspoon ground cumin

½ teaspoon chili powder

½ teaspoon red pepper flakes

¼ teaspoon dried oregano

1 tablespoon lime juice

1. Heat oil in a large skillet over medium-high heat. Add garlic, jalapeño, and onion and cook until softened, about 4 minutes. Stir in rice and cook 1 more minute.
2. Add remaining ingredients and stir to combine. Bring to a boil, cover, and reduce heat to low. Simmer 15 minutes or until rice is tender. Remove from heat and allow to cool 30 minutes.
3. Divide evenly into six airtight containers. Cover and store in refrigerator until ready to eat, up to 1 week.
4. When ready to serve, transfer to a skillet, cover, and cook over low heat 5 minutes or until heated through.

Chickpea Curry with Basmati Rice

SERVES 6

Per Serving:

Calories	308
Fat	5g
Sodium	563mg
Carbohydrates	54g
Fiber	11g
Sugar	9g
Protein	12g

WHAT IS BASMATI RICE?

Basmati rice is grown in the Himalayas, India, and Pakistan. It's higher in carbs and calories than regular white rice, but also has a bit more protein. Unlike other rice, it expands in length, rather than width, when it's cooked. It has a light, fluffy texture and a slightly nutty taste. If you don't have basmati rice on hand, you can use any other rice in its place, but it's worth adding to your pantry.

This curry is excellent with basmati rice, but you can also serve it with brown rice or naan bread, if you prefer. If you want to cut carbs, you can also skip the rice altogether or use cauliflower rice instead. Finely chopped parsley or cilantro would be a welcome addition as a garnish before serving.

1 (15-ounce) can tomato sauce
1 cup light coconut milk
⅓ cup red curry paste
1 teaspoon garam masala
½ teaspoon ground cumin
½ teaspoon sea salt
¼ teaspoon ground black pepper
¼ teaspoon red pepper flakes
2 (15-ounce) cans chickpeas, drained and rinsed
2 tablespoons lime juice
3 cups cooked basmati rice

1. Combine tomato sauce, coconut milk, curry paste, garam masala, cumin, salt, black pepper, and red pepper flakes in a large saucepan over medium-high heat. Cook 2 minutes.
2. Stir in chickpeas and reduce heat to low. Cook 10 minutes or until chickpeas are softened and heated through. Stir in lime juice. Remove from heat.
3. Scoop ½ cup rice into each of six airtight containers. Scoop equal portions of chickpea curry into each container. Cover and store in refrigerator until ready to eat, up to 1 week.
4. When ready to serve, transfer to a skillet, cover, and cook over low heat 5 minutes or until heated through.

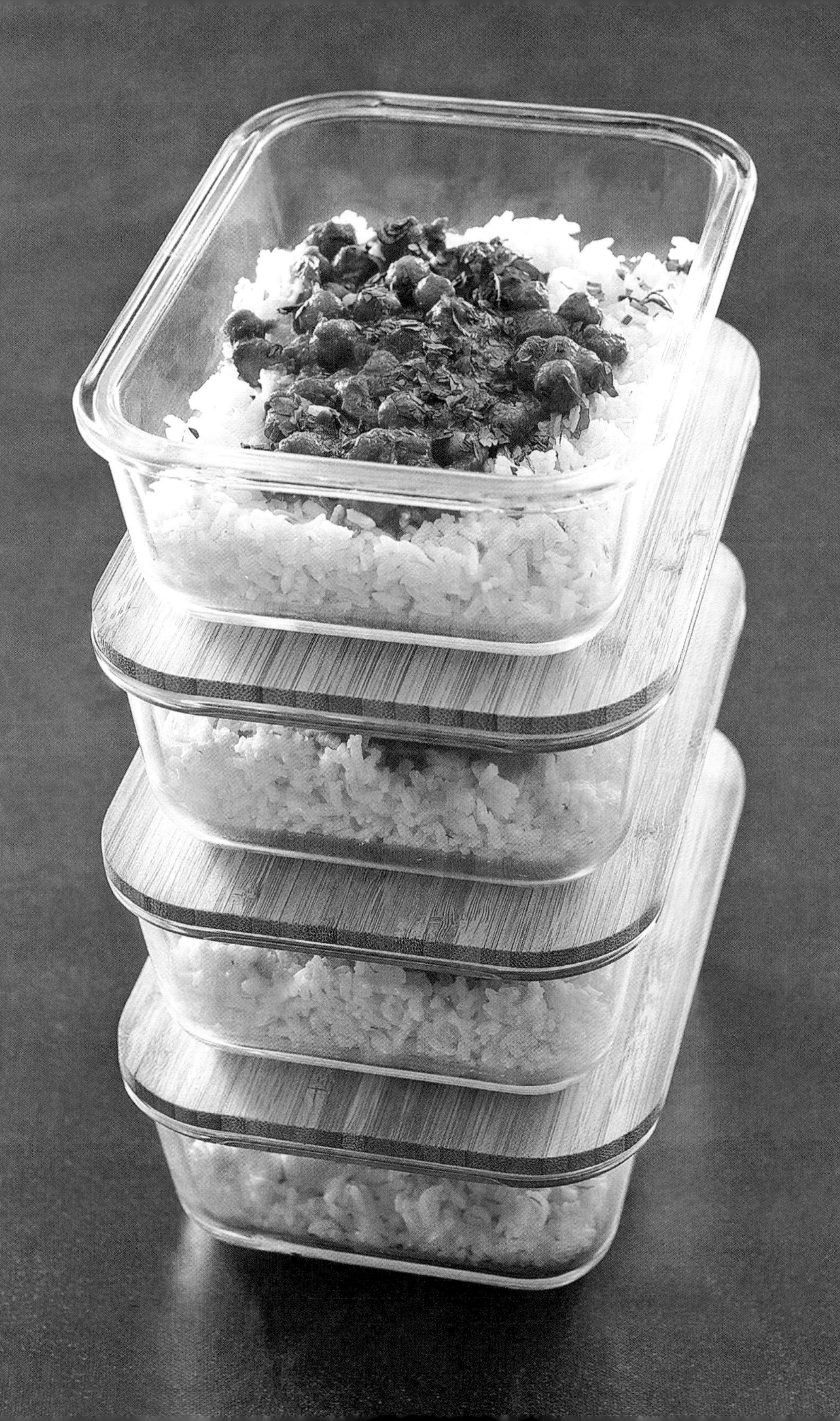

Tex-Mex Quinoa

SERVES 6

Per Serving:

Calories	241
Fat	3g
Sodium	480mg
Carbohydrates	42g
Fiber	8g
Sugar	6g
Protein	12g

If you don't have a pressure cooker, you can make this Tex-Mex Quinoa on the stovetop instead. Mix all the ingredients together, cook over medium heat for 15 minutes, then cover the pan and let the quinoa sit for 5 minutes before fluffing with a fork

1 cup vegetable broth

1 cup quinoa, rinsed well

1 cup frozen peas

1 cup frozen sweet corn kernels

1 (15-ounce) can black beans, drained and rinsed

1 large green bell pepper, seeded and finely chopped

1 (1.3-ounce) packet Siete Taco Seasoning

½ cup no-sugar-added salsa

1. Combine broth and quinoa in pressure cooker. Stir in peas, corn, beans, bell pepper, and taco seasoning. Pour salsa on top.
2. Close the lid, set to manual/high pressure cook/manual, and set time for 1 minute. When time is up, allow pressure to release naturally.
3. Carefully open lid and stir. Allow to cool 20 minutes.
4. Divide evenly into six airtight containers. Cover and store in refrigerator until ready to eat, up to 1 week.
5. When ready to serve, transfer to a skillet, cover, and cook over low heat 5 minutes or until heated through.

Zucchini Bean Burrito Boats

If you want to slightly drop the carbs in this recipe, you can swap out the rice for quinoa, or omit the starch all together. Omitting the cheese will help reduce the fat content.

SERVES 6

Per Serving:

Calories	204
Fat	8g
Sodium	550mg
Carbohydrates	22g
Fiber	5g
Sugar	3g
Protein	11g

3 large zucchini, halved lengthwise

2 teaspoons avocado oil

1 medium green bell pepper, seeded and diced

¼ cup minced red onion

1 small jalapeño, seeded and minced

1 (15-ounce) can black beans, drained and rinsed

½ cup cooked brown rice

¾ cup no-sugar-added salsa

2 teaspoons ground cumin

1 teaspoon chili powder

1 teaspoon sea salt

⅓ cup chopped fresh cilantro

¾ cup shredded Cheddar cheese

1. Preheat oven to 400°F.
2. Use a spoon to seed zucchini and hollow out center to create a well. Arrange zucchini cut-side up in a 9" × 13" baking dish.
3. Heat oil in a large skillet over medium heat. Add bell pepper and onion and cook until peppers start to soften, about 5 minutes. Stir in jalapeño and cook another 3 minutes.
4. Add remaining ingredients, except cheese, and mix well. Cook until heated through, about 5 minutes.
5. Scoop filling into each zucchini half and sprinkle cheese on top. Cover dish with aluminum foil and bake 25 minutes or until zucchini softens and filling is bubbly. Remove foil and bake 5 minutes more. Remove from oven and allow to cool 20 minutes.
6. Transfer zucchini boats to each of six airtight containers. Cover and store in refrigerator until ready to eat, up to 1 week.
7. When ready to serve, transfer to a baking sheet and broil on low 3 minutes or until cheese is bubbly and zucchini is heated through.

Tofu Teriyaki

SERVES 6

Per Serving:

Calories	279
Fat	8g
Sodium	511mg
Carbohydrates	39g
Fiber	5g
Sugar	8g
Protein	12g

When prepping your tofu, make sure you pat it dry and then cut evenly. Keeping all the cubes the same size will ensure more even cooking and a better result.

3 tablespoons cornstarch, divided

18 ounces extra-firm tofu, cut into 1" cubes

2 teaspoons avocado oil

1 small yellow onion, peeled and finely diced

3 cloves garlic, peeled and minced

2 teaspoons shredded fresh ginger

½ cup coconut aminos

2 tablespoons Swerve brown sweetener

2 tablespoons rice vinegar

1 teaspoon toasted sesame oil

2 tablespoons water

6 cups steamed broccoli florets

3 cups cooked white rice

1 tablespoon sesame seeds

1 medium scallion, chopped

1. Place 2 tablespoons cornstarch in a shallow dish. Pat tofu dry and dredge each piece in a thin layer of cornstarch. Set aside.
2. Heat avocado oil in a large skillet over medium-high heat. Add tofu to hot pan and cook 10 minutes or until tofu is golden brown, turning to brown all sides. Remove from pan and set aside.
3. Add onion to hot pan and cook 4 minutes. Stir in garlic and ginger and cook another 1 minute. Add coconut aminos, sweetener, vinegar, and sesame oil and stir.
4. Whisk remaining 1 tablespoon cornstarch and water in a small bowl until smooth, then stir into sauce. Cook 4 minutes or until sauce starts to thicken. Add cooked tofu to pan and toss to coat. Cook 1 more minute, then remove from heat.
5. Scoop 1 cup broccoli and ½ cup rice into each of six airtight containers. Divide tofu evenly into containers. Sprinkle sesame seeds and scallion on top of tofu. Cover and store in refrigerator until ready to eat, up to 1 week.
6. Serve cold, or transfer to a skillet, cover, and cook over low heat 5 minutes or until heated through.

Mediterranean Stuffed Peppers

The natural sweetness of red bell peppers complements this dish nicely, but if you want to drop the carbs a bit, you can use green bell peppers in their place. You can also use zucchini boats instead of bell peppers if you want to switch things up.

SERVES 6

Per Serving:

Calories	334
Fat	3g
Sodium	582mg
Carbohydrates	59g
Fiber	16g
Sugar	6g
Protein	17g

6 red bell peppers, tops cut off, seeded

2 teaspoons extra-virgin olive oil

1 small yellow onion, peeled and minced

2 cloves garlic, peeled and minced

1 (15-ounce) can chickpeas drained and rinsed

3 cups cooked brown lentils

3 cups cooked sprouted brown rice

½ cup chopped roasted red peppers

¼ cup tomato sauce

1 tablespoon tomato paste

1 teaspoon dried oregano

1 teaspoon sea salt

½ teaspoon ground black pepper

½ cup vegetable broth

1. Preheat oven to 350°F.
2. Stand bell peppers up in a 9" × 13" baking dish.
3. Heat oil in a large skillet over medium heat. Add onion and cook 4 minutes. Stir in garlic and cook 1 minute. Add chickpeas, lentils, and rice and stir to combine.
4. Stir in remaining ingredients and bring to a slow boil. Reduce heat to low and cook 5 minutes or until some liquid has dissolved and mixture is heated through.
5. Scoop equal parts mixture into each bell pepper. Cover baking dish with aluminum foil and bake 40 minutes. Remove foil and bake 5 minutes more or until peppers are softened. Remove from oven and allow to cool 30 minutes.
6. Transfer stuffed peppers to each of six airtight containers. Cover and store in refrigerator until ready to eat, up to 1 week.
7. When ready to serve, transfer to a small baking dish and cook at 300°F 15 minutes or until heated through.

Kidney Bean Burgers

SERVES 4

Per Serving:

Calories	122
Fat	0g
Sodium	841mg
Carbohydrates	23g
Fiber	6g
Sugar	3g
Protein	7g

THE MACROS IN KIDNEY BEANS

Kidney beans have a beautiful macronutrient profile that makes them easy to fit into most meals. Each ½ cup kidney beans contains 22 grams of carbohydrates (7 grams of which come from fiber), 8 grams of protein, and 0.5 grams of fat. Kidney beans are also rich in vitamins, minerals, and antioxidants, making them a nutrient-dense choice for a macro diet.

These Kidney Bean Burgers are super easy to make and packed with protein. You can eat them as is, throw them on top of your favorite salad for a quick protein boost, or serve them on your favorite bun that fits into your macros.

1 (15-ounce) can kidney beans, drained and rinsed

¼ cup minced red onion

2 tablespoons Tessemae's Unsweetened Ketchup

1 teaspoon garlic powder

1 teaspoon onion powder

¾ teaspoon sea salt

¾ cup cooked sprouted brown rice

1. Preheat oven to 400°F. Line a baking sheet with parchment paper.
2. Put beans in a large bowl and mash them. Add remaining ingredients to bowl and mix well.
3. Divide mixture into four equal portions and form each portion into a patty. Arrange patties on prepared baking sheet.
4. Bake 20 minutes, carefully flipping once halfway through cooking. Remove from oven and allow to cool 20 minutes.
5. Transfer patties to each of four airtight containers. Cover and store in refrigerator until ready to eat, up to 1 week.
6. When ready to serve, transfer to a skillet, cover, and cook over medium heat 5 minutes or until heated through.

Chickpea Burgers

Because these burgers are baked and not pan-fried, they're lower in fat. If you have some fat allowance, you can top them with sliced avocado or guacamole or make a spicy mayonnaise sauce.

SERVES 6

Per Serving:

Calories	252
Fat	2g
Sodium	773mg
Carbohydrates	44g
Fiber	15g
Sugar	3g
Protein	15g

2 cups grated zucchini

2 teaspoons sea salt, divided

2 (15-ounce) cans chickpeas, drained and rinsed

½ cup peeled grated carrots

¼ cup minced red onion

3 cloves garlic, peeled and minced

¼ cup chickpea flour

2 tablespoons sriracha

1 teaspoon ground cumin

1. Preheat oven to 400°F. Line a baking sheet with parchment paper.
2. Put grated zucchini in a strainer and sprinkle with 1 teaspoon salt. Let sweat 15 minutes.
3. While zucchini is sweating, put chickpeas in a large mixing bowl and mash with a fork. Add remaining ingredients, including remaining 1 teaspoon salt.
4. Transfer zucchini to a cheesecloth or nut bag and squeeze out as much excess liquid as you can. Add zucchini to chickpea mixture and mix well.
5. Divide mixture into six equal portions and shape each portion into a patty. Arrange patties on prepared baking sheet.
6. Bake 20 minutes, carefully flipping once while cooking. Remove from oven and allow to cool 20 minutes.
7. Transfer patties to each of six airtight containers. Cover and store in refrigerator until ready to eat, up to 1 week.
8. When ready to serve, transfer to a skillet, cover, and cook over medium heat 5 minutes or until heated through.

Portobello Fajitas

SERVES 6

Per Serving:

Calories	221
Fat	3g
Sodium	337mg
Carbohydrates	43g
Fiber	5g
Sugar	8g
Protein	6g

PROTEIN IN PORTOBELLO MUSHROOMS

Because of their rich flavor and meaty texture, portobello mushrooms are often used as a vegan or vegetarian replacement for meat. They don't have the same amount of protein—1 cup of chopped mushroom has about 2.2 grams—but they're still satisfying. If you want to add some protein to a meal that has portobello mushrooms, beans or chickpeas are always an excellent (and fiber-rich) choice.

Instead of brown rice, you can serve these Portobello Fajitas with soft tortillas. Any option that fits into your macros will work, but Siete makes a grain-free version if you're trying to stay away from corn or gluten.

3 medium sweet potatoes, peeled and cut into 3" strips

5 large portobello mushrooms, cut into 3" strips

1 large red bell pepper, seeded and cut into 3" strips

1 large red onion, peeled and sliced

2 teaspoons extra-virgin olive oil

1 (1.3-ounce) packet Siete Taco Seasoning

3 cups cooked sprouted brown rice

1. Preheat oven to 400°F. Line a baking sheet with parchment paper.
2. Add sweet potatoes, mushrooms, bell pepper, and onion to a large mixing bowl. Drizzle oil over vegetables and toss to coat. Sprinkle taco seasoning on top and toss again.
3. Spread vegetables out in a single layer on prepared baking sheet. Roast 30 minutes or until sweet potato is tender. Remove from oven and set aside.
4. Put ½ cup cooked brown rice in each of six airtight containers. Divide vegetable mixture evenly into each container. Cover and store in refrigerator until ready to eat, up to 1 week.
5. When ready to serve, transfer to a skillet, cover, and cook over medium heat 5 minutes or until heated through.

Spicy Vegetarian Pad Thai

If you can't have peanut butter, you can use equal amounts of almond butter in its place, but it will drop the protein a bit. If you want a high-protein substitution, you can use one of the nut butter flavors from Nuts 'n More or RXBAR.

SERVES 6

Per Serving:

Calories	404
Fat	12g
Sodium	723mg
Carbohydrates	64g
Fiber	3g
Sugar	3g
Protein	10g

FOR SAUCE

- ⅓ cup coconut aminos
- 3 tablespoons no-sugar-added creamy peanut butter
- 2 tablespoons Swerve brown sweetener
- 2 tablespoons lime juice
- 2 tablespoons sriracha
- 2 tablespoons red curry paste
- 1 tablespoon toasted sesame oil

FOR NOODLES

- 1 (14-ounce) box rice noodles
- 1 teaspoon toasted sesame oil
- ½ cup peeled sliced shallots
- 1 large jalapeño, seeded and diced
- 5 cloves garlic, peeled and minced
- 3 large eggs, lightly beaten
- 2 tablespoons chopped scallions
- 3 tablespoons chopped peanuts

1. To make Sauce: Whisk all ingredients in a small bowl until smooth. Set aside.
2. To make Noodles: Bring a large pot of water to a boil over high heat. Add rice noodles, reduce heat to medium-high, and cook 4 minutes or according to package instructions. Drain and set aside.
3. Heat oil in a wok or large skillet over medium-high heat. Add shallots, jalapeño, and garlic and cook until jalapeño starts to soften, about 5 minutes. Add eggs and scramble. Stir in noodles and Sauce. Remove from heat and allow to cool 30 minutes.
4. Divide evenly into six airtight containers. Sprinkle scallions and peanuts on top, cover, and refrigerate until ready to eat, up to 1 week.
5. When ready to serve, transfer to a skillet, cover, and cook over medium heat 5 minutes or until heated through.

LESSEN THE SPICE

If you like the flavor of jalapeños but you wish you could make them a little less spicy, there's a trick for that. Aside from removing the seeds (a lot of the spice is in the seeds), you can soak the jalapeños in a 3:1 water and white vinegar solution for 1 hour before adding them to your recipes. Make sure you cut them in half or quarters first. The flesh has to be exposed to the vinegar solution for it to work.

Lentil Taco Soup

SERVES 6

Per Serving:

Calories	237
Fat	3g
Sodium	970mg
Carbohydrates	38g
Fiber	12g
Sugar	13g
Protein	14g

LOVE ON LENTILS

Like beans, lentils are a beautifully balanced legume that can help you meet your macro goals. Each ½ cup of lentils offers 20 grams of carbohydrates (7.8 grams of which come from fiber), 9 grams of protein, and less than 0.5 grams of fat. Lentils are also an excellent source of B vitamins, magnesium, potassium, iron, and zinc.

Make sure you watch the lentils as they cook and take them off the heat when they're soft but not too mushy. They'll soften a little more as they sit in the refrigerator, and if you overcook them, they'll lose some of their texture as the week goes on.

1 teaspoon avocado oil

1 medium yellow onion, peeled and chopped

4 cloves garlic, peeled and minced

1 (1.3-ounce) packet Siete Taco Seasoning

1 medium green bell pepper, seeded and finely diced

1 small jalapeño, seeded and finely diced

4 cups vegetable broth

1 (15-ounce) can petite-diced tomatoes, including juice

1 cup dried brown lentils, rinsed

1 (15-ounce) can black beans, drained and rinsed

1 cup frozen sweet corn kernels

1. Heat oil in a large stockpot or Dutch oven over medium-high heat. Add onion and cook 4 minutes. Add garlic and cook 1 minute. Sprinkle taco seasoning on top and stir to combine. Add bell pepper and jalapeño to pot and cook 2 minutes.
2. Pour broth and tomatoes with juice into pot and stir. Add lentils and cook 25 minutes or until lentils are soft but not mushy. Stir in beans and corn and cook 5 minutes. Remove from heat and allow to cool 20 minutes.
3. Divide evenly into six airtight containers. Cover and store in refrigerator up to 1 week, or in freezer up to 3 months, until ready to eat.
4. When ready to serve, transfer to a skillet, cover, and cook over medium heat 5 minutes or until heated through.

CHAPTER 9

Side Dishes

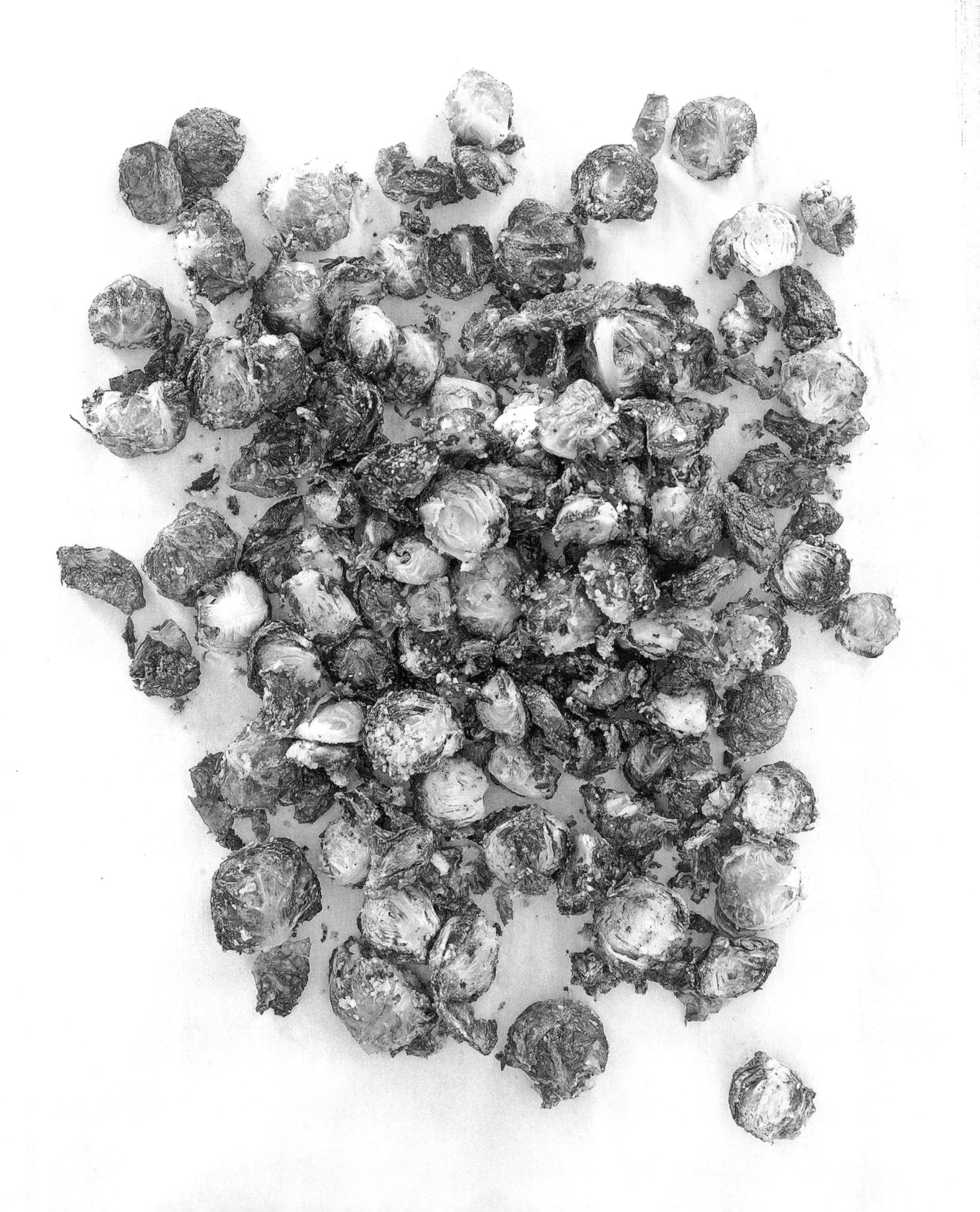

Air-Fried Parmesan Garlic Brussels Sprouts

If you don't have an air fryer, you can make these Brussels sprouts in the oven. Prep the Brussels sprouts, lay them out in a single layer on a baking sheet, and roast them at 400°F for 20–25 minutes or until fork-tender.

SERVES 6

Per Serving:

Calories	140
Fat	6g
Sodium	494mg
Carbohydrates	15g
Fiber	7g
Sugar	7g
Protein	7g

2 tablespoons unsalted grass-fed butter, melted
1 tablespoon extra-virgin olive oil
1 teaspoon minced garlic
2 pounds Brussels sprouts, trimmed and halved
1 teaspoon sea salt
½ teaspoon ground black pepper
1 teaspoon garlic powder
½ teaspoon onion powder
⅓ cup grated Parmesan cheese

1. Preheat air fryer to 400°F.
2. Add butter, oil, and garlic to a large bowl and whisk together. Add Brussels sprouts and toss to coat evenly. Sprinkle remaining ingredients on top and toss again to coat.
3. Transfer Brussels sprouts to ungreased air fryer basket and fry 20 minutes, gently tossing Brussels sprouts once during cooking. Remove from air fryer and allow to cool 30 minutes.
4. Divide evenly into six airtight containers. Cover and store in refrigerator until ready to eat, up to 1 week.
5. When ready to serve, transfer to a skillet and cook over medium heat 5 minutes or until heated through.

BENEFITS OF BRUSSELS

Brussels sprouts belong to the *Brassica oleracea* family of cruciferous vegetables, a category they share with broccoli, cabbage, cauliflower, kale, and collard greens. One thing these vegetables have in common, aside from their health benefits, is their characteristic odor. That odor comes from a sulfur-containing compound called glucosinolate. Although glucosinolate is stinky, it's a phytochemical that protects you from cancer, reduces your risk of heart attack, and staves off inflammatory diseases.

Everything Bagel Roasted Potatoes

SERVES 6

Per Serving:

Calories	67
Fat	2g
Sodium	160mg
Carbohydrates	11g
Fiber	1g
Sugar	1g
Protein	1g

These Everything Bagel Roasted Potatoes are so easy to make, and go well with any main proteins. You can pair them with eggs for a quick and easy breakfast, or add them right into your meal prep containers alongside any beef, pork, poultry, or seafood dish.

1 pound baby potatoes, cut into quarters

2 teaspoons avocado oil

1 tablespoon everything bagel seasoning

1. Preheat oven to 425°F. Line a baking sheet with parchment paper.
2. Add potatoes to a large bowl and drizzle oil on top. Toss to coat. Sprinkle seasoning on top and toss to coat again.
3. Spread potatoes out on prepared baking sheet. Bake 30 minutes or until potatoes are tender and starting to turn golden brown. Remove from oven and allow to cool 30 minutes.
4. Divide evenly into six airtight containers. Cover and refrigerate until ready to eat, up to 1 week.
5. When ready to serve, heat in air fryer at 325°F or under a broiler on low 5 minutes (watching carefully) until crispy.

RESISTANT STARCH FOR THE WIN

White potatoes have developed a bad rap over the years, but they can actually be really good for you, especially when properly worked into a balanced macro diet. White potatoes are rich in resistant starch, a type of carbohydrate that is resistant to digestion. Because of this, resistant starch has little to no effect on your blood sugar. It does, however, act as a prebiotic, feeding the good bacteria in your gut and contributing to healthy digestion and all of the other benefits that come with a healthy gut.

Ranch-Roasted Cauliflower

It's worth stocking your cabinet with Flavor God Ranch Topper, but if you don't have it and you want to make this recipe anyway, you can replace it with a homemade ranch spice blend (parsley, dried dill, dried chives, garlic powder, onion powder, salt, and pepper) or another ranch shaker of your choosing.

SERVES 6

Per Serving:

Calories	66
Fat	5g
Sodium	287mg
Carbohydrates	4g
Fiber	1g
Sugar	1g
Protein	1g

6 cups cauliflower florets

2 tablespoons avocado oil

1 teaspoon lemon juice

2 teaspoons Flavor God Ranch Topper

½ teaspoon sea salt

¼ teaspoon ground black pepper

1. Preheat oven to 375°F. Line a baking sheet with parchment paper.
2. Put cauliflower in a large bowl and drizzle oil and lemon juice on top. Toss to coat evenly. Sprinkle spices on top of cauliflower and toss again.
3. Arrange cauliflower in a single layer on prepared baking sheet. Bake 30 minutes or until cauliflower is tender and starting to brown. Remove from oven and allow to cool 30 minutes.
4. Divide evenly into six airtight containers. Cover and refrigerate until ready to eat, up to 1 week.
5. When ready to serve, heat in air fryer at 325°F or in oven on a low broil 5 minutes (watching carefully) until crispy.

Baked Parmesan Turnip Fries

These fries are just as satisfying as the "real" thing but with a fraction of the carbohydrates. If you're trying to keep your carbs low, these will become your go-to side dish or easy-to-grab snack. Enjoy it with no-sugar-added ketchup as a dip if it fits your macros!

SERVES 6

Per Serving:

Calories	91
Fat	3g
Sodium	398mg
Carbohydrates	13g
Fiber	3g
Sugar	7g
Protein	3g

2½ pounds turnips, peeled and cut into 3" sticks
1 tablespoon avocado oil
1 teaspoon garlic powder
1 teaspoon paprika
½ teaspoon sea salt
½ teaspoon ground black pepper
¼ cup grated Parmesan cheese

1. Preheat oven to 425°F. Line two baking sheets with parchment paper.
2. Put turnip fries in a large bowl and drizzle with oil. Toss to coat. Sprinkle garlic powder, paprika, salt, and pepper on top. Toss to coat again. Sprinkle Parmesan on top.
3. Spread turnips out in a single layer on prepared baking sheets. Bake 20 minutes, flip fries over, and bake another 20 minutes or until crispy. Remove from oven and allow to cool 30 minutes.
4. Divide evenly into six airtight containers. Cover and refrigerate until ready to eat, up to 1 week.
5. When ready to serve, heat in air fryer at 325°F or under a broiler on low 5 minutes (watching carefully) until crispy.

TURNIPS VERSUS POTATOES

Turnips are often used as a lower-carb substitute for potatoes in side dishes, soups, and casseroles. For comparison, 1 cup of diced turnips has about 8 grams of carbohydrates (3 grams of which come from fiber), while 1 cup of diced potatoes packs in 31 grams of carbohydrates (3 grams of fiber). Turnips are prepared in the same way but have a slightly sweeter flavor. However, when they're seasoned and cooked, you can hardly tell.

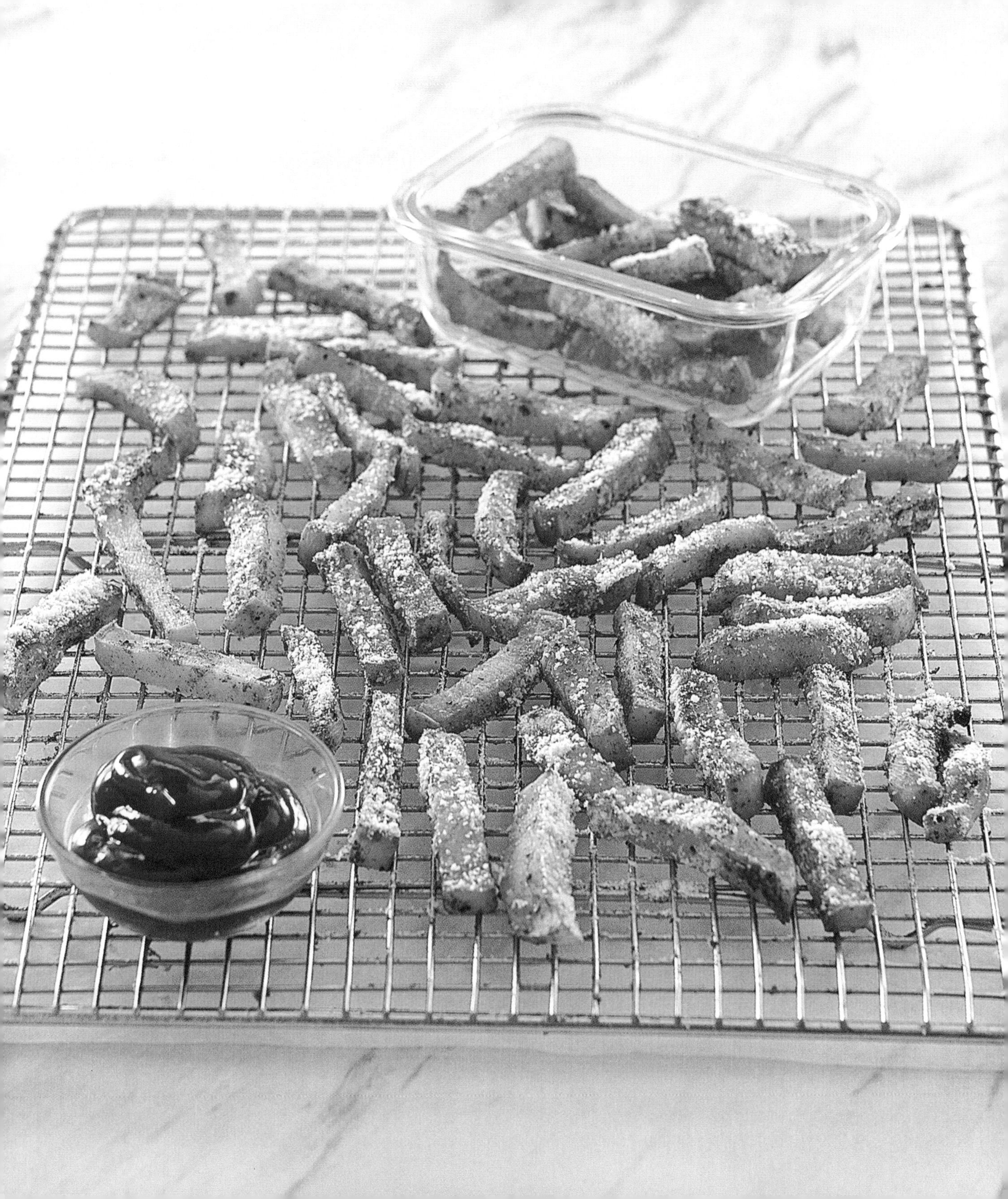

Cheesy Cauliflower Casserole

SERVES 6

Per Serving:

Calories	101
Fat	5g
Sodium	340mg
Carbohydrates	6g
Fiber	2g
Sugar	2g
Protein	7g

It's easy to tweak the macros in this recipe by scaling back on the cheese or using different types of Greek yogurt. You can also add a few potatoes if you have some carbs to spare and want a denser texture.

1 large cauliflower head, cut into florets
¾ cup shredded Cheddar cheese, divided
⅓ cup 2% plain Greek yogurt
1 teaspoon garlic powder
½ teaspoon smoked paprika
½ teaspoon sea salt
¼ teaspoon ground black pepper

1. Preheat oven to 375°F. Spray a 9" × 9" baking dish with avocado oil cooking spray and set aside.
2. Bring a large pot of water to a boil over high heat. Add cauliflower and cook until tender, about 10 minutes. Drain.
3. Transfer cauliflower to a food processor and add ½ cup Cheddar, yogurt, and spices. Process until smooth, about 2 minutes.
4. Transfer puréed cauliflower to prepared baking dish and sprinkle remaining ¼ cup Cheddar on top. Bake 20 minutes or until cheese is melted and casserole is hot and bubbly. Remove from oven and allow to cool 1 hour.
5. Divide evenly into six airtight containers. Cover and store in refrigerator until ready to eat, up to 1 week.
6. When ready to serve, transfer to a skillet and cook over medium heat 5 minutes or until heated through.

Chickpea and Feta Salad

If you need to scale back on fat, you can eliminate the feta cheese or olives from this recipe. Because they're both fairly high in salt, you may need to adjust the spices accordingly, so taste it as you go!

SERVES 6

Per Serving:

Calories	321
Fat	22g
Sodium	843mg
Carbohydrates	22g
Fiber	7g
Sugar	2g
Protein	9g

FOR DRESSING

⅓ cup extra-virgin olive oil
2 tablespoons red wine vinegar
1 tablespoon lemon juice
1 teaspoon dried parsley
½ teaspoon sea salt
¼ teaspoon ground black pepper

FOR SALAD

2 (15-ounce) cans chickpeas, drained and rinsed
1 medium cucumber, cut into coins and then quartered
½ small red onion, peeled and thinly sliced
½ cup sliced kalamata olives
½ cup crumbled feta cheese
½ cup halved cherry tomatoes
½ teaspoon sea salt
¼ teaspoon ground black pepper

1. To make Dressing: Whisk all ingredients in a small bowl until smooth.
2. To make Salad: Add all ingredients to a large bowl and gently stir. Pour Dressing on top and toss to coat.
3. Divide evenly into six airtight containers. Cover and store in refrigerator until ready to eat, up to 1 week. Serve cold.

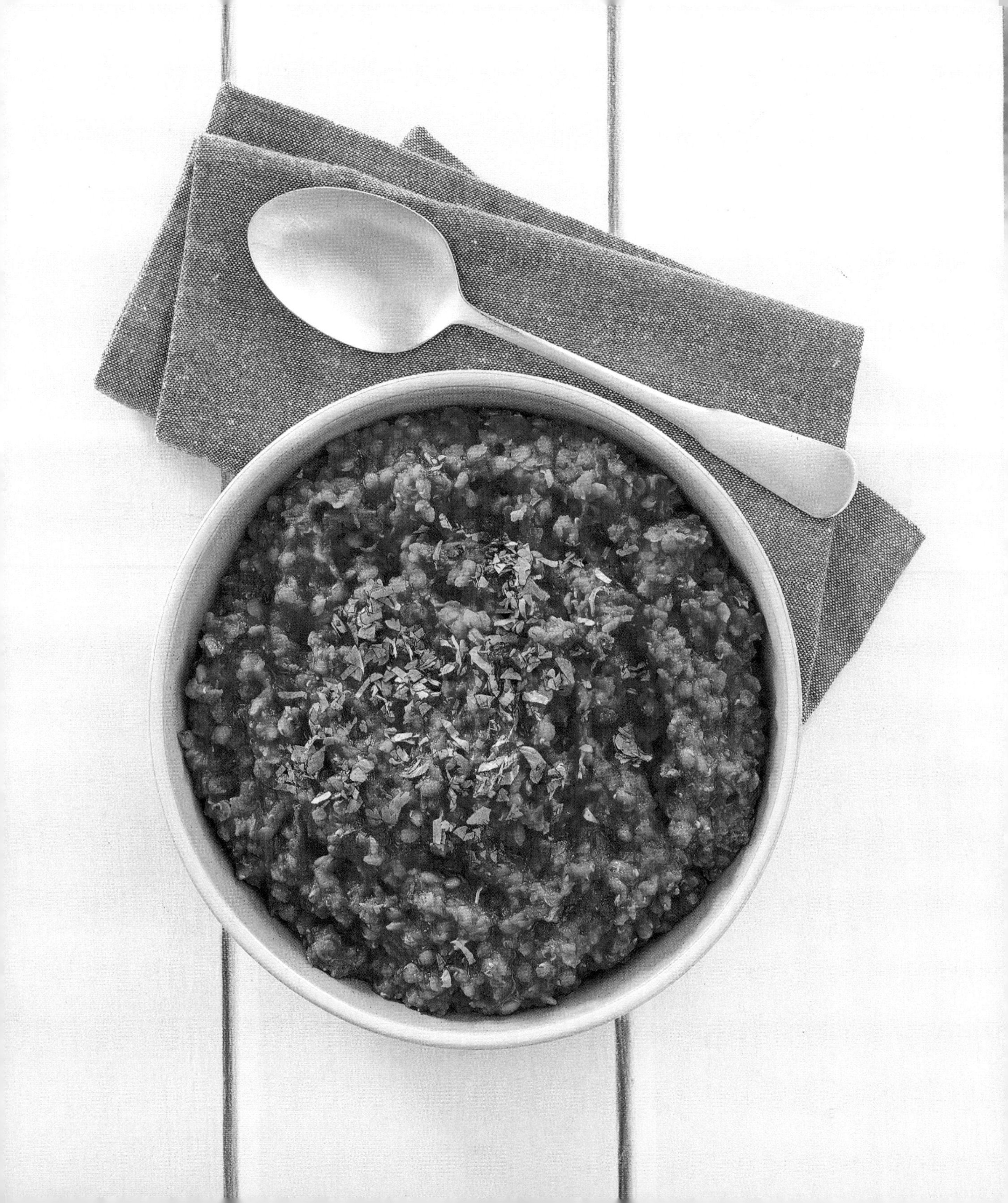

Spicy Red Lentils

It's worth the extra effort to find a harissa spice blend or a harissa paste to make this recipe. If you can't, you can use a combination of smoked paprika, ground cumin, ground coriander, caraway seeds, garlic powder, and salt, but you will lose some of the heat. Feel free to add finely chopped herbs like parsley or cilantro as a garnish before serving.

SERVES 6

Per Serving:

Calories	218
Fat	2g
Sodium	27mg
Carbohydrates	34g
Fiber	16g
Sugar	3g
Protein	15g

2 teaspoons extra-virgin olive oil
1 medium yellow onion, peeled and diced
3 cloves garlic, peeled and minced
2 tablespoons harissa spice blend
¼ teaspoon cayenne pepper
3 tablespoons tomato paste
1 tablespoon diced fire-roasted green chiles
1½ cups dried red lentils, rinsed
2 cups chicken broth

1. Heat oil in a large stockpot or Dutch oven over medium-high heat. Add onion and cook 4 minutes. Add garlic and cook another 2 minutes or until onion is translucent and garlic is fragrant.
2. Add harissa, cayenne pepper, tomato paste, and green chiles and stir to heat through. Stir in lentils to coat.
3. Pour in broth, making sure lentils are fully covered, and stir. Reduce heat to low and simmer 20 minutes. Remove from heat and allow to cool 20 minutes.
4. Divide evenly into six airtight containers. Cover and store in refrigerator until ready to eat, up to 1 week.
5. When ready to serve, transfer to a skillet, cover, and cook over medium heat 5 minutes or until heated through.

WHAT IS HARISSA?

Harissa is a red chile paste that originates in Tunisia and is common in North African and Middle Eastern cooking. In addition to various aromatic spices and a sweet, yet smoky flavor, it packs some serious heat. If you don't have harissa, you can use some hot sauce in its place, but it won't be an exact substitute. Adding the real thing to your pantry is highly recommended.

Sweet and Sour Roasted Cabbage

SERVES 6

Per Serving:

Calories	96
Fat	3g
Sodium	421mg
Carbohydrates	14g
Fiber	7g
Sugar	10g
Protein	3g

GO RAW

You may have heard honey is good for you, but most of the health benefits are attributed to raw honey, which comes directly from the beehive. It's not pasteurized or filtered (only strained), so it retains all of its nutrients and also contains the bee pollen, which is removed from other honeys. Bee pollen contains over 250 health-promoting substances, including vitamins, minerals, amino acids, essential fatty acids, and antioxidants. It's been linked to decreased inflammation, improved liver function, and better heart health. It can also help ward off seasonal allergies.

The blend of different kinds of cabbage adds a little something special to this recipe, but if you want to make meal prep a bit easier, you can use one kind of cabbage instead.

1 tablespoon extra-virgin olive oil

1 tablespoon red wine vinegar

2 teaspoons raw honey

1 small head green cabbage, cored and chopped

1 small head red cabbage, cored and chopped

1 small sweet onion, peeled and sliced thinly

1 teaspoon sea salt

1. Preheat oven to 400°F. Spray a 9" × 13" baking dish with avocado oil cooking spray.
2. Whisk together oil, vinegar, and honey in a small bowl. Set aside.
3. Add both cabbages and onion to prepared baking dish. Sprinkle with salt and toss to coat.
4. Bake 30 minutes or until cabbage is tender, stirring halfway through cooking. Remove from oven and immediately pour oil mixture on top. Toss to coat. Allow to cool 30 minutes.
5. Divide evenly into six airtight containers. Cover and store in refrigerator until ready to eat, up to 1 week. Serve cold.

Autumn Vegetable Hash

If pumpkin isn't in season, you can replace it with extra sweet potatoes. You can also sneak in white potatoes or cubed turnips if you're looking for a lower-carb alternative. If you want to cut the fat, lose the bacon (or drop down to one piece for just a little bit of smoky flavor).

SERVES 6

Per Serving:

Calories	85
Fat	1g
Sodium	363mg
Carbohydrates	15g
Fiber	4g
Sugar	7g
Protein	4g

2 slices no-sugar-added bacon

1 large sweet potato, peeled and diced

2 cups peeled cubed pumpkin

2 cups Brussels sprouts, trimmed and halved

2 medium carrots, peeled and diced

1 medium yellow onion, peeled and chopped

2 teaspoons ground sage

1 teaspoon dried thyme

1 teaspoon sea salt

1. Preheat oven to 400°F. Line a baking sheet with parchment paper.
2. In a small skillet, cook bacon over medium-high heat 6 minutes or until almost crispy. Transfer bacon with a slotted spoon to a paper towel–lined plate, reserving bacon fat in pan. Roughly chop bacon.
3. Add sweet potato, pumpkin, Brussels sprouts, carrots, onion, and 1 tablespoon bacon fat to a large bowl. Toss to combine and evenly coat. Sprinkle spices on top and toss again to coat.
4. Spread vegetables out in a single layer on prepared baking sheet. Bake 45 minutes or until vegetables are softened and starting to crisp. Sprinkle bacon on top and bake another 2 minutes to crisp bacon. Remove from oven and allow to cool 30 minutes.
5. Divide evenly into six airtight containers. Cover and store in refrigerator until ready to eat, up to 1 week.
6. When ready to serve, transfer to a skillet, cover, and cook over medium heat 5 minutes or until heated through.

Mexican Street Corn

SERVES 6

Per Serving:

Calories	362
Fat	33g
Sodium	505mg
Carbohydrates	14g
Fiber	2g
Sugar	4g
Protein	3g

WHAT IS MEXICAN STREET CORN?

If you've never had the pleasure of enjoying Mexican street corn, also known as *elote*, you don't know what you're missing. Street vendors in Mexico serve corn covered with some combination of butter, mayonnaise, chili powder, cayenne pepper, and Cotija cheese—a salty, crumbly authentic treat. Traditionally, Mexican Street Corn is served on the cob, but using canned corn turns it into an easy-to-prep side dish.

If you've ever been to Mexico, you know what a treat authentic Mexican street corn is. This version mimics the same great flavors but with less fat—and in an easier-to-eat preparation that can be made up to a week in advance.

1½ teaspoons unsalted grass-fed butter

1 (15-ounce) can whole kernel corn, drained and patted dry

¼ cup 2% plain Greek yogurt

1 tablespoon Tessemae's Mayonnaise

2 teaspoons lime juice

2 teaspoons chopped fresh cilantro

1 teaspoon chili powder

½ teaspoon sea salt

1. Heat butter in a large skillet over medium-high heat. Add corn and cook until it starts to char, about 7 minutes.
2. While corn is cooking, add remaining ingredients to a large mixing bowl and whisk to combine. Add charred corn to mixture and stir to coat. Allow to cool 30 minutes.
3. Divide evenly into six airtight containers. Cover and refrigerate until ready to eat, up to 1 week.
4. Serve cold.

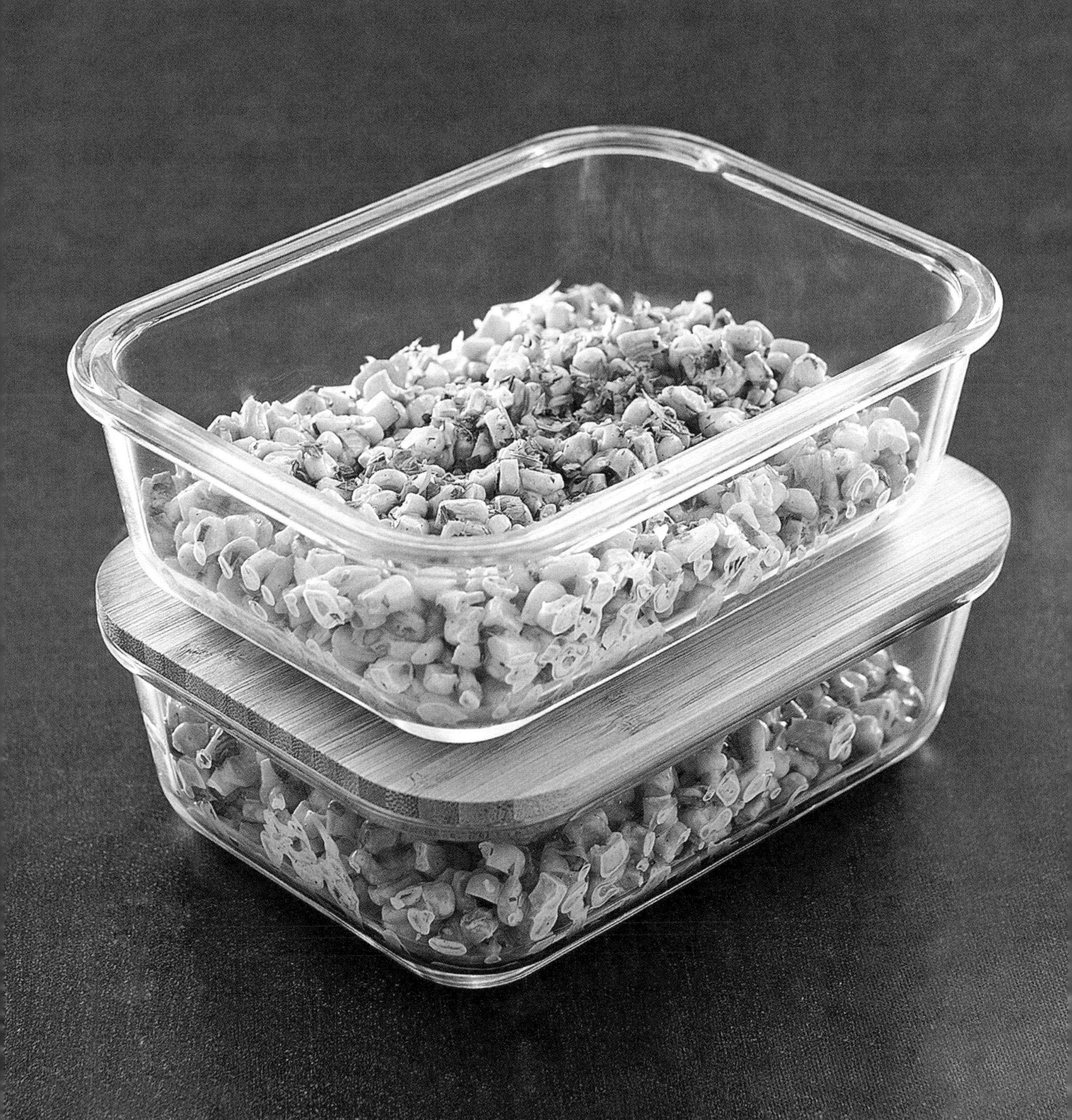

White Bean and Tomato Salad

SERVES 6

Per Serving:

Calories	268
Fat	12g
Sodium	474mg
Carbohydrates	23g
Fiber	11g
Sugar	2g
Protein	15g

This White Bean and Tomato Salad tastes even better after sitting in the refrigerator for a couple days, so don't be afraid to prep a big batch in advance.

- ¼ cup extra-virgin olive oil
- 2 tablespoons lemon juice
- 1 tablespoon apple cider vinegar
- ½ teaspoon minced garlic
- ½ teaspoon sea salt
- ¼ teaspoon ground black pepper
- 2 (15-ounce) cans cannellini beans, drained and rinsed
- ¼ cup halved cherry tomatoes
- 2 tablespoons minced red onion
- 3 tablespoons crumbled feta cheese
- ¼ cup chopped fresh parsley

1. Whisk together oil, lemon juice, vinegar, garlic, salt, and pepper in a large bowl.
2. Add remaining ingredients and stir well, making sure ingredients are mixed and coated.
3. Divide evenly into six airtight containers. Cover and refrigerate until ready to eat, up to 1 week. Serve cold.

Caesar Salad Brussels Sprouts

Just like a salad, these Caesar Salad Brussels Sprouts are delicious cold right out of the refrigerator, but if you want to heat them up before eating them, air fry them for 2–3 minutes.

SERVES 6

Per Serving:

Calories	109
Fat	8g
Sodium	523mg
Carbohydrates	6g
Fiber	3g
Sugar	3g
Protein	3g

12 ounces Brussels sprouts, trimmed and halved

2 tablespoons extra-virgin olive oil

1 teaspoon sea salt

½ teaspoon ground black pepper

½ teaspoon garlic powder

⅓ cup Tessemae's Creamy Caesar Dressing

3 tablespoons grated Parmesan cheese

1. Preheat air fryer to 375°F.
2. Add Brussels sprouts to a large bowl. Drizzle with oil and sprinkle salt, pepper, and garlic powder on top. Toss to evenly coat.
3. Transfer Brussels sprouts to preheated, ungreased air fryer basket 15 minutes or until Brussels sprouts are tender and slightly browned, tossing once during cooking.
4. When Brussels sprouts are done, remove from air fryer and return to bowl. Add dressing and Parmesan to bowl and toss to coat.
5. Divide evenly into six airtight containers. Cover and store in refrigerator until ready to eat, up to 1 week.

Broccoli Fried Rice

SERVES 6

Per Serving:

Calories	122
Fat	2g
Sodium	314mg
Carbohydrates	22g
Fiber	3g
Sugar	2g
Protein	4

This Broccoli Fried Rice combines fiber, slow-acting carbs, and tons of vitamin C and vitamin K, thanks to the broccoli. If you want to lower the carbs, you can swap out the brown rice for cauliflower rice. To increase protein without a major change to the fat content, add some lean ground turkey.

2 teaspoons toasted sesame oil

1 teaspoon minced fresh ginger

1 large head broccoli, roughly chopped

3 cups cooked brown rice

2 tablespoons coconut aminos

½ teaspoon sea salt

¼ teaspoon ground black pepper

¼ teaspoon red pepper flakes

1. Heat oil in a large skillet or wok over medium-high heat. Add ginger and cook 1 minute. Add broccoli and cook 5 minutes or until it starts to soften. Stir in rice and cook another 3 minutes to heat it through. Remove from heat and stir in coconut aminos and spices. Allow to cool 30 minutes.
2. Divide evenly into six airtight containers. Cover and store in refrigerator until ready to eat, up to 1 week.
3. When ready to serve, spray a pan with avocado oil cooking spray and cook on medium for 5 minutes or until heated through.

Brussels Slaw

The raisins add a sweet touch and a welcome chewy texture to this Brussels Slaw, but if you want to cut some carbs, you can leave them out. You can also play around with different amounts of honey or other low-carb sweeteners.

SERVES 6

Per Serving:

Calories	350
Fat	27g
Sodium	637mg
Carbohydrates	19g
Fiber	5g
Sugar	13g
Protein	8g

½ cup light olive oil

¼ cup red wine vinegar

1 tablespoon Dijon mustard

2 teaspoons raw honey

1 teaspoon sea salt

½ teaspoon ground black pepper

1 pound very thinly sliced Brussels sprouts

½ cup crushed walnuts

¾ cup crumbled feta cheese

1 medium Honeycrisp apple, cored and thinly sliced

¼ cup raisins

1. Whisk oil, vinegar, mustard, honey, salt, and pepper in a small bowl until smooth.
2. Add remaining ingredients to a large bowl and mix well. Add dressing and toss to coat evenly.
3. Divide evenly into six airtight containers. Cover and store in refrigerator until ready to eat, up to 1 week. Serve cold.

Butternut and Cauliflower Mash

SERVES 6

Per Serving:

Calories	94
Fat	5g
Sodium	425mg
Carbohydrates	10g
Fiber	3g
Sugar	3g
Protein	2g

BETA-CAROTENE IN BUTTERNUT SQUASH

Butternut squash is loaded with antioxidants, including beta-carotene, the pigment that also gives carrots, sweet potatoes, and pumpkin their signature orange hue. Beta-carotene protects your vision, supports your immune system, and keeps your skin healthy. Some studies show that beta-carotene can also protect your lungs and brain from decline as you age.

This Butternut and Cauliflower Mash literally goes with everything. Pair it with rotisserie chicken for an almost effortless prepped meal, or combine it with the Firecracker Chicken (see recipe in Chapter 5) to add a little kick to your week.

1 large head cauliflower, cut into florets

1 small butternut squash, peeled and cut into 1" cubes

2 tablespoons Nutiva Buttery Flavor Coconut Oil, melted

1 tablespoon light coconut milk

1 teaspoon minced garlic

1 teaspoon ground sage

1 teaspoon sea salt

1. Bring a large pot of water to a boil. Add cauliflower and squash and cook until soft, about 8 minutes. Drain and transfer to a food processor.
2. Add oil and coconut milk and purée until smooth, about 4 minutes, stopping to scrape down the sides of the bowl as necessary. Add garlic, sage, and salt and briefly process to combine, about 30 seconds.
3. Divide evenly into six airtight containers. Cover and refrigerate until ready to eat, up to 1 week.
4. When ready to serve, add to a saucepan, cover and heat over medium heat 5 minutes, stirring occasionally, or until cooked through.

Cinnamon Sweet Potatoes

Raw honey gives these Cinnamon Sweet Potatoes a sticky-sweet flavor and texture, but if you want to cut the carbs back a little bit, you can replace it with ChocZero Maple-Flavored Syrup for a similar result.

SERVES 6

Per Serving:

Calories	99
Fat	3g
Sodium	261mg
Carbohydrates	17g
Fiber	3g
Sugar	5g
Protein	1g

1 teaspoon raw honey

1 tablespoon avocado oil

1 teaspoon ground cinnamon

¼ teaspoon ground nutmeg

4 medium sweet potatoes, peeled and cut into 1" cubes

½ teaspoon flaked sea salt

¼ teaspoon ground black pepper

1. Preheat oven to 375°F. Line a baking sheet with parchment paper.
2. Add honey, oil, cinnamon, and nutmeg to a large bowl and whisk until smooth. Add sweet potatoes and toss to coat evenly.
3. Spread potatoes out in an even layer on prepared baking sheet. Sprinkle salt and pepper on top. Bake 30 minutes or until potatoes are soft and starting to turn golden brown, gently stirring halfway through cooking. Remove from oven and allow to cool 30 minutes.
4. Divide evenly into six airtight containers. Cover and refrigerate until ready to eat, up to 1 week.
5. Serve cold, or heat in a skillet over medium heat 5 minutes or until cooked through.

Spicy Black Bean Salad

Using black beans gives this dish a nice, hearty flavor, but you can switch things up by using chickpeas instead, or a combination of both types of beans. And since there's no cooking, it comes together in minutes no matter which beans you choose!

SERVES 6

Per Serving:

Calories	194
Fat	3g
Sodium	431mg
Carbohydrates	33g
Fiber	8g
Sugar	3g
Protein	9g

2 (15-ounce) cans black beans, drained and rinsed
1 cup fire-roasted corn kernels
¼ cup minced red onion
¼ cup minced fresh cilantro
¼ cup fresh lime juice
1 tablespoon extra-virgin olive oil
1 teaspoon garlic powder
1 teaspoon chili powder
½ teaspoon ground cumin
½ teaspoon smoked paprika
¼ teaspoon sea salt

1. Combine beans, corn, onion, and cilantro in a large bowl.
2. In a small bowl, whisk together remaining ingredients. Pour over bean mixture.
3. Divide evenly into six airtight containers. Cover and refrigerate until ready to eat, up to 1 week. Serve cold.

BENEFITS OF BLACK BEANS

Black beans are high in total carbohydrates, but much of those carbs come in the form of soluble fiber, which doesn't have an impact on your blood sugar. Because of this, beans are considered a low-glycemic food. Some studies show that when you eat black beans with rice, the beans can blunt the blood sugar spike that rice can have on its own. The soluble fiber in beans has also been linked to lower risk of heart disease and better management of inflammation.

Baked Greek Cauliflower Rice

Using frozen cauliflower rice makes it easy to whip this side dish up, but if you want it a little less runny, you can make your own fresh cauliflower rice by passing a head of cauliflower through the shredding attachment of a food processor.

SERVES 6

Per Serving:

Calories	114
Fat	9g
Sodium	865mg
Carbohydrates	5g
Fiber	3g
Sugar	3g
Protein	4g

1 tablespoon extra-virgin olive oil

1 small red onion, peeled and minced

⅓ cup chopped roasted red peppers

⅓ cup chopped kalamata olives

2 (10-ounce) packages frozen cauliflower rice

1 tablespoon Greek seasoning

½ cup crumbled feta cheese, divided

⅓ cup sliced scallions

1. Preheat oven to 375°F. Spray a 9" × 13" baking dish with avocado oil cooking spray.
2. Heat oil in a large skillet over medium-high heat. Add onion and cook until translucent, about 5 minutes. Reduce heat to medium, add red peppers and olives, and cook until warmed through, about 2 minutes.
3. Add cauliflower rice and cook until clumps are broken up, about 4 minutes. Sprinkle Greek seasoning on top and continue to cook until rice is tender, about 5 more minutes. Remove from heat and stir in ¼ cup feta and scallions.
4. Transfer mixture to prepared baking dish and spread out evenly. Sprinkle remaining ¼ cup feta on top. Bake 30 minutes or until heated through and bubbly. Remove from oven and allow to cool 30 minutes.
5. Divide evenly into six airtight containers. Cover and refrigerate until ready to eat, up to 1 week.
6. When ready to serve, heat in a skillet over medium heat 5 minutes or until heated through.

High-Protein Caprese Pasta Salad

SERVES 6

Per Serving:

Calories	182
Fat	5g
Sodium	327mg
Carbohydrates	22g
Fiber	6g
Sugar	4g
Protein	12g

Thanks to its chickpea base, Banza pasta is high in protein—but it also contains a considerable amount of carbohydrates. If you can't fit it into your macros, or you just prefer a different macro ratio, you can use your favorite type of pasta or pasta substitute, like spaghetti squash, in its place.

1 (8-ounce) box Banza rotini

2 tablespoons pesto

2 teaspoons balsamic vinegar

½ teaspoon sea salt

¼ teaspoon ground black pepper

1 cup halved grape tomatoes

½ cup chopped fresh basil

½ cup quartered mozzarella pearls

1. Bring a medium pot of water to a boil over high heat. Add pasta and cook according to the package instructions. Drain.
2. While pasta is cooking, add pesto, vinegar, salt, and pepper to a small bowl and whisk until smooth.
3. Add cooked pasta to a large bowl, along with tomatoes, basil, and mozzarella. Stir to combine. Drizzle pesto mixture on top and toss to coat. Allow to cool 30 minutes.
4. Divide evenly into six airtight containers. Cover and refrigerate until ready to eat, up to 1 week. Serve cold.

Cauliflower "Potato" Salad

If you have some extra carbs to spare, you can combine cauliflower and potatoes in this salad instead of using only cauliflower to add some different textures.

SERVES 6

Per Serving:

Calories	184
Fat	16g
Sodium	373mg
Carbohydrates	5g
Fiber	2g
Sugar	2g
Protein	5g

1 large head cauliflower, cut into florets

¼ cup minced red onion

3 cloves garlic, peeled and minced

1 medium stalk celery, finely chopped

3 large hard-boiled eggs, peeled and roughly chopped

½ cup Tessemae's Mayonnaise

1 tablespoon white vinegar

1 teaspoon mustard powder

½ teaspoon sea salt

½ teaspoon garlic powder

½ teaspoon dried dill

¼ teaspoon paprika

¼ teaspoon ground black pepper

1. Bring a large pot of water to a boil over high heat. Add cauliflower and reduce heat to medium-high. Cook 6 minutes or until cauliflower is tender but not overcooked. Drain and allow to cool 10 minutes.
2. Transfer cauliflower to a large bowl. Add onion, garlic, celery, and eggs and gently stir.
3. Whisk remaining ingredients in a small bowl until smooth. Pour dressing on top and toss to coat evenly.
4. Divide into six airtight containers. Cover and store in refrigerator until ready to eat, up to 1 week. Serve cold.

CHAPTER 10

Snacks and Appetizers

Snickers Baked Oatmeal

SERVES 6

Per Serving (2 squares):

Calories	303
Fat	13g
Sodium	303mg
Carbohydrates	40g
Fiber	26g
Sugar	1g
Protein	8g

This Snickers Baked Oatmeal will become a go-to for snack, breakfast, and even dessert. If you want to make it more portable, you can pour the batter into a muffin tin lined with paper or silicone liners. Just reduce the cooking time by 10 minutes or so.

2 cups gluten-free rolled oats

1 tablespoon ground flaxseeds

1 teaspoon baking powder

½ teaspoon sea salt

1½ cups unsweetened vanilla almond milk

⅓ cup no-sugar-added creamy peanut butter

½ cup ChocZero Maple-Flavored Syrup

2 teaspoons vanilla extract

¼ cup chopped peanuts

⅓ cup Lily's stevia-sweetened chocolate chips

1. Preheat oven to 350°F. Line a 9" × 9" baking dish with parchment paper.
2. Combine oats, flaxseeds, baking powder, and salt in a large bowl.
3. Combine remaining ingredients in a separate large bowl. Add wet ingredients to dry ingredients and fold to combine.
4. Pour mixture into prepared dish. Bake 40 minutes or until a toothpick inserted in center comes out clean. Allow to cool completely, about 1 hour.
5. Cut into twelve squares. Transfer to an airtight container and store at room temperature until ready to eat, up to 2 weeks.

GLUTEN IN OATS

Oats are naturally gluten-free, but most oats in the US are processed in the same facilities as the gluten-containing grains, wheat, barley, and rye. Because of this, many packaged oats are contaminated with gluten and no longer considered gluten-free. If you want gluten-free oats, check the package and make sure you see a gluten-free label or certification.

Rice Cake PB&J

It might not seem ideal to meal prep rice cakes, but when you let them sit in the refrigerator with the strawberry preserves, the flavors meld together so well. And it makes it really easy to grab a balanced snack when you're in a major rush.

SERVES 4

Per Serving:

Calories	147
Fat	6g
Sodium	2mg
Carbohydrates	18g
Fiber	3g
Sugar	1g
Protein	5g

4 tablespoons natural no-sugar-added peanut butter

8 brown rice cakes

8 teaspoons no-sugar-added strawberry preserves

2 teaspoons hemp seeds

1. Spread 1 tablespoon peanut butter on each of 4 rice cakes. Top each with 2 teaspoons preserves. Sprinkle ½ teaspoon hemp seeds over preserves. Top with remaining 4 rice cakes.
2. Transfer to an airtight container and store in refrigerator until ready to eat, up to 4 days. Serve cold or at room temperature.

Shredded Chicken and Bacon Dip

You can pair this dip with anything you want. Gluten-free crackers are a great option if you have some room in your carb allowance. If you want to keep it low-carb, try raw zucchini slices or celery stalks.

SERVES 6

Per Serving:

Calories	382
Fat	23g
Sodium	385mg
Carbohydrates	0g
Fiber	0g
Sugar	0g
Protein	41g

2 (12-ounce) cans cooked chicken breast

1 tablespoon chopped scallions

6 slices no-sugar-added bacon, cooked and roughly chopped

½ cup shredded Cheddar cheese

1 teaspoon minced garlic

½ cup Tessemae's Mayonnaise

1. Combine all ingredients in a large bowl.
2. Divide evenly into six airtight containers. Cover and store in refrigerator up to 1 week, until ready to eat. Serve cold.

Chocolate Chip Pumpkin Protein Muffins

YIELDS 12 MUFFINS

Per Serving (1 muffin):

Calories	133
Fat	3g
Sodium	37mg
Carbohydrates	14g
Fiber	2g
Sugar	2g
Protein	12g

If you don't have oat flour, you can grind gluten-free rolled oats in a food processor until a powdered flour forms. You can also use regular chocolate chips in place of Lily's, which are sweetened with stevia, but you'll have to adjust your macros accordingly.

1¼ cups oat flour

½ cup Tera's Whey vanilla protein powder

1 teaspoon ground cinnamon

½ teaspoon pumpkin pie spice

1 teaspoon baking powder

1 teaspoon baking soda

1 cup pumpkin purée

¾ cup 2% plain Greek yogurt

2 large eggs

½ cup Lily's stevia-sweetened chocolate chips

1. Preheat oven to 350°F. Line a twelve-cup muffin tin with paper or silicone liners.
2. Combine oat flour, protein powder, cinnamon, pumpkin pie spice, baking powder, and baking soda in a large bowl.
3. Add pumpkin purée, yogurt, and eggs to a separate large bowl and lightly whisk to combine. Fold pumpkin mixture into dry mixture and stir until just combined. Stir in chocolate chips.
4. Scoop equal amounts of batter into each muffin cup. Bake 20 minutes or until a toothpick inserted in center comes out clean. Allow to cool completely, about 1 hour.
5. Transfer to an airtight container. Store at room temperature until ready to eat, up to 2 weeks.

PLANT-BASED PROTEIN POWDER

There are many different protein powder options out there, and any of them will work in the recipes in this book that call for protein powder. If you don't consume whey, which has most of the lactose removed and is highly digestible, your best bet is to use hemp protein in its place. Hemp is not only a complete protein; it also has a nice nutty flavor that complements sweet dishes, and it blends in well. The fat content will be a few grams higher, though, so make sure you're accounting for that when you're calculating your macros.

Maple Peanut Butter Oat Bars

These four-ingredient oat bars are delicious and easy to put together since they don't require any baking. Just make sure you store them in the refrigerator. If you leave them at room temperature, they'll fall apart.

YIELDS 12 BARS

Per Serving (1 bar):

Calories	214
Fat	10g
Sodium	6mg
Carbohydrates	25g
Fiber	13g
Sugar	2g
Protein	7g

1 cup no-sugar-added crunchy peanut butter
½ cup ChocZero Maple-Flavored Syrup
2¾ cups gluten-free rolled oats
2 tablespoons ground flaxseeds

1. Line an 8" × 8" baking dish with parchment paper.
2. Add peanut butter to a small saucepan over low heat. Stir until melted, about 3 minutes. Add maple syrup and stir until smooth, about 1 minute. Remove from heat and set aside.
3. Combine oats and flaxseeds in a medium bowl. Stir into peanut butter mixture.
4. Transfer mixture to prepared baking dish and press down evenly. Refrigerate until set, about 1 hour.
5. Remove set mixture from dish and cut into twelve bars. Transfer to an airtight container, cover, and store in refrigerator until ready to eat, up to 2 weeks.

GRIND AS YOU GO

Flaxseeds are high in healthy fats, which is a good thing. But like other fat-rich foods, they can go rancid when stored for an extended period. Because of this, it's best to buy whole flaxseeds and grind them with a coffee grinder or a food processor when you want to use them. It's a little extra work, but it will ensure that you're always enjoying fresh flaxseeds with the highest nutrient profile.

Spicy Baked Chickpeas

SERVES 6

Per Serving:

Calories	179
Fat	5g
Sodium	465mg
Carbohydrates	25g
Fiber	9g
Sugar	0g
Protein	9g

These Spicy Baked Chickpeas are the perfect snack for those days when you need something to satisfy your craving for some crunch. And unlike other popular snack foods, they're full of protein and actually help fill you up.

1 tablespoon paprika

2 teaspoons sea salt

2 teaspoons granulated garlic

1 teaspoon ground black pepper

1 teaspoon onion powder

1 teaspoon cayenne pepper

1 teaspoon dried oregano

2 (15-ounce) cans chickpeas, drained, rinsed, and patted dry

2 tablespoons avocado oil

1. Preheat oven to 400°F. Line a baking sheet with parchment paper.
2. Combine paprika, salt, garlic, black pepper, onion powder, cayenne pepper, and oregano in a medium bowl.
3. Toss chickpeas with oil in a large bowl. Sprinkle seasoning mixture over chickpeas and toss to coat evenly.
4. Spread seasoned chickpeas out on prepared baking sheet. Roast 45 minutes, turning once while baking. Remove from oven and allow to cool completely, about 30 minutes.
5. Divide chickpeas evenly into six sandwich bags and seal. Store at room temperature until ready to eat, up to 1 week.

PAT DRY BEFORE YOU ROAST

Whenever you're roasting chickpeas, make sure you drain and rinse them and then pat them as dry as possible. The drier the chickpeas are when they go into the oven, the crispier your finished snack will be. If you want to make the chickpeas even crunchier, you can peel off the skins after you rinse them (it's easier than it sounds).

Zucchini Cheddar Bites

Psyllium husk helps hold these Zucchini Cheddar Bites together and helps keep your gut regular. You can omit it if you don't have it, but it's an ingredient worth adding to your pantry.

SERVES 6

Per Serving (3 bites):

Calories	109
Fat	8g
Sodium	287mg
Carbohydrates	2g
Fiber	0g
Sugar	1g
Protein	7g

1½ cups grated zucchini
½ teaspoon sea salt
3 large eggs, lightly beaten
1 cup almond meal
2 tablespoons psyllium husk
1 tablespoon dried parsley
1 teaspoon granulated garlic
1 teaspoon paprika
1 cup shredded Cheddar cheese

1. Preheat oven to 375°F. Line a baking sheet with parchment paper.
2. Put zucchini in a strainer and sprinkle with salt. Set aside and let sweat 10 minutes.
3. Transfer zucchini to a cheesecloth or nut bag and squeeze out excess liquid. Put zucchini in a large bowl and add remaining ingredients. Mix until combined.
4. Form into eighteen equal-sized balls and arrange on prepared baking sheet. Press down on each ball to slightly flatten.
5. Bake 20 minutes or until zucchini bites start to turn golden brown. Remove from oven and allow to cool 30 minutes.
6. Transfer to an airtight container, cover, and store in refrigerator until ready to eat, up to 1 week.
7. When ready to serve, reheat at 300°F 10 minutes or until warmed through, then broil on high 1-2 minutes until crispy.

WHAT IS PSYLLIUM HUSK?

Psyllium husk is a type of soluble fiber that supports proper digestion. It's often used to treat chronic constipation, but it has a smooth, gentle effect rather than the harsh stimulant effect of some laxatives. Although each tablespoon of psyllium husk has 8 grams of carbohydrates, all of those carbohydrates are in the form of fiber, so it has no effect on your blood sugar.

Protein Gra-No-La

SERVES 6

Per Serving:

Calories	714
Fat	46g
Sodium	213mg
Carbohydrates	34g
Fiber	20g
Sugar	2g
Protein	40g

This oat-less granola is lower in carbs than traditional granola but has plenty of healthy fats to help you reach your fat goals for the day. Take it with you for a snack or put some on top of yogurt. You can make a large batch and store extras in an airtight container.

1 cup whole almonds
1 cup whole cashews
1 cup whole pumpkin seeds
1 cup whole sunflower seeds
2 tablespoons whole flaxseeds
¼ cup Nutiva Buttery Flavor Coconut Oil
⅓ cup ChocZero Maple-Flavored Syrup
2 teaspoons ground cinnamon
½ teaspoon flaked sea salt
1 teaspoon vanilla extract
¾ cup Lily's stevia-sweetened chocolate chips

1. Preheat oven to 275°F. Lightly spray a baking sheet with avocado oil cooking spray.
2. Add almonds, cashews, pumpkin seeds, sunflower seeds, and flaxseeds to a food processor and lightly pulse about 20 seconds until nuts are slightly chopped. Don't over overprocess.
3. Add oil, maple syrup, cinnamon, and salt to a large saucepan over low heat. Melt and cook 5 minutes, stirring frequently. Remove from heat and stir in vanilla.
4. Fold in nut mixture and stir to coat evenly.
5. Spread mixture out on prepared baking sheet. Bake 25 minutes or until granola starts to turn golden brown. Remove from oven and sprinkle chocolate chips evenly on top.
6. Allow to cool 1 hour. Break into chunks and transfer equal amounts to each of six airtight containers or sandwich bags. Store at room temperature until ready to eat, up to 2 weeks.

Cheesy Black Bean Dip

This Cheesy Black Bean Dip is high in protein and fiber, so it's as filling as it is delicious. You can serve it with grain-free tortilla chips, celery stalks, raw zucchini slices, or crackers—whatever fits into your macros.

SERVES 4

Per Serving:

Calories	219
Fat	10g
Sodium	537mg
Carbohydrates	19g
Fiber	7g
Sugar	1g
Protein	13g

2 teaspoons extra-virgin olive oil

1 (15-ounce) can black beans, drained and rinsed

1⁄3 cup 2% plain Greek yogurt

3⁄4 teaspoon ground cumin

1⁄2 teaspoon sea salt

1⁄2 teaspoon chili powder

1 clove garlic, peeled and minced

11⁄2 tablespoons lime juice

3⁄4 cup shredded pepper Jack cheese

1. Preheat oven to 400°F.
2. Add all ingredients, except cheese, to a food processor and process 1 minute or until smooth. Spoon mixture into an 8" × 8" baking pan. Sprinkle cheese on top.
3. Bake 20 minutes or until dip is hot and bubbly and cheese is melted. Remove from oven and allow to cool 30 minutes.
4. Divide mixture evenly into four airtight containers. Cover and store in refrigerator until ready to eat, up to 1 week.
5. When ready to serve, heat in a saucepan over low heat 3 minutes or until heated through.

Cheesy Protein Popcorn

SERVES 6

Per Serving:

Calories	177
Fat	8g
Sodium	421mg
Carbohydrates	13g
Fiber	2g
Sugar	1g
Protein	13g

A COMPLETE PROTEIN

Nutritional yeast is a deactivated strain of yeast, usually *Saccharomyces cerevisiae,* that's often used as a cheese powder substitute in vegan cooking. In addition to the savory flavor it adds to dishes, it's also loaded with fiber and various vitamins and minerals, like vitamin B_{12} and folic acid. It also contains all nine essential amino acids, which makes it a complete protein—and a tasty way to add protein to your meals. Just sprinkle it on anything where you need a boost.

Unflavored whey protein is the "secret" ingredient in this protein popcorn, but you can use any protein powder—dairy or non—that you like. For best results, just make sure it's high quality, free of artificial ingredients, and unflavored.

⅓ cup Bragg's nutritional yeast
⅓ cup Tera's Whey plain unsweetened protein powder
1 teaspoon sea salt
3 tablespoons Nutiva Buttery Flavor Coconut Oil
½ cup organic popcorn kernels

1. Combine nutritional yeast, protein powder, and salt in a large container with a lid.
2. Heat oil in a large saucepan over medium heat. Add a handful of popcorn kernels to oil. Once kernels begin to pop, about 5 minutes, add remaining kernels. Cover saucepan and shake to coat kernels with oil.
3. As kernels begin to pop, shake pan every few seconds to move kernels around and prevent popped corn from burning. When popping slows down to 2 seconds between pops, remove from heat and transfer popcorn to container with yeast mixture.
4. Cover and shake vigorously to coat evenly. Transfer 2 cups popcorn to each of six airtight containers. Store at room temperature until ready to eat, up to 1 week.

Cauliflower Arancini

If you've ever had arancini, or Italian rice balls, you already know what a delight they are. This version packs all the same flavor but with considerably fewer carbs, thanks to using cauliflower in place of rice.

SERVES 6

Per Serving:

Calories	180
Fat	13g
Sodium	764mg
Carbohydrates	7g
Fiber	3g
Sugar	4g
Protein	9g

- 2 teaspoons avocado oil
- 4½ cups cauliflower rice
- 1½ teaspoons sea salt, divided
- 1½ cups no-sugar-added pizza sauce, divided
- 1 cup part-skim shredded mozzarella cheese
- 2 large eggs
- ½ cup almond meal
- 1 teaspoon garlic powder
- 1 teaspoon onion powder
- 1 teaspoon dried parsley
- ½ teaspoon ground black pepper
- 2 tablespoons grated Parmesan cheese

1. Preheat air fryer to 400°F.
2. Heat oil in a large skillet over medium heat. Add cauliflower, 1 teaspoon salt, and ¾ cup pizza sauce and stir to combine. Cook 8 minutes or until cauliflower is tender and some liquid from sauce has evaporated.
3. Remove from heat and stir in mozzarella. Allow mixture to cool 20 minutes or until cool enough to handle.
4. While cauliflower mixture is cooling, lightly beat eggs in a small bowl. In a separate small bowl, combine almond meal, garlic powder, onion powder, parsley, pepper, Parmesan, and remaining ½ teaspoon salt.
5. Divide cauliflower mixture into twelve equal balls. Carefully dip each ball in egg and then evenly coat with almond meal mixture.
6. Lightly spray each ball with avocado oil cooking spray and arrange in ungreased air fryer basket. Fry 10 minutes or until golden brown on the outside, flipping each ball halfway through the cooking process.
7. Remove from air fryer and allow to cool 30 minutes. Transfer two arancini to each of six airtight containers. Add 2 tablespoons remaining pizza sauce to each of six small containers. Place small containers in large containers, cover, and store in refrigerator until ready to eat, up to 1 week.
8. When ready to serve, heat 2 minutes in air fryer or 30 seconds in microwave and serve with pizza sauce.

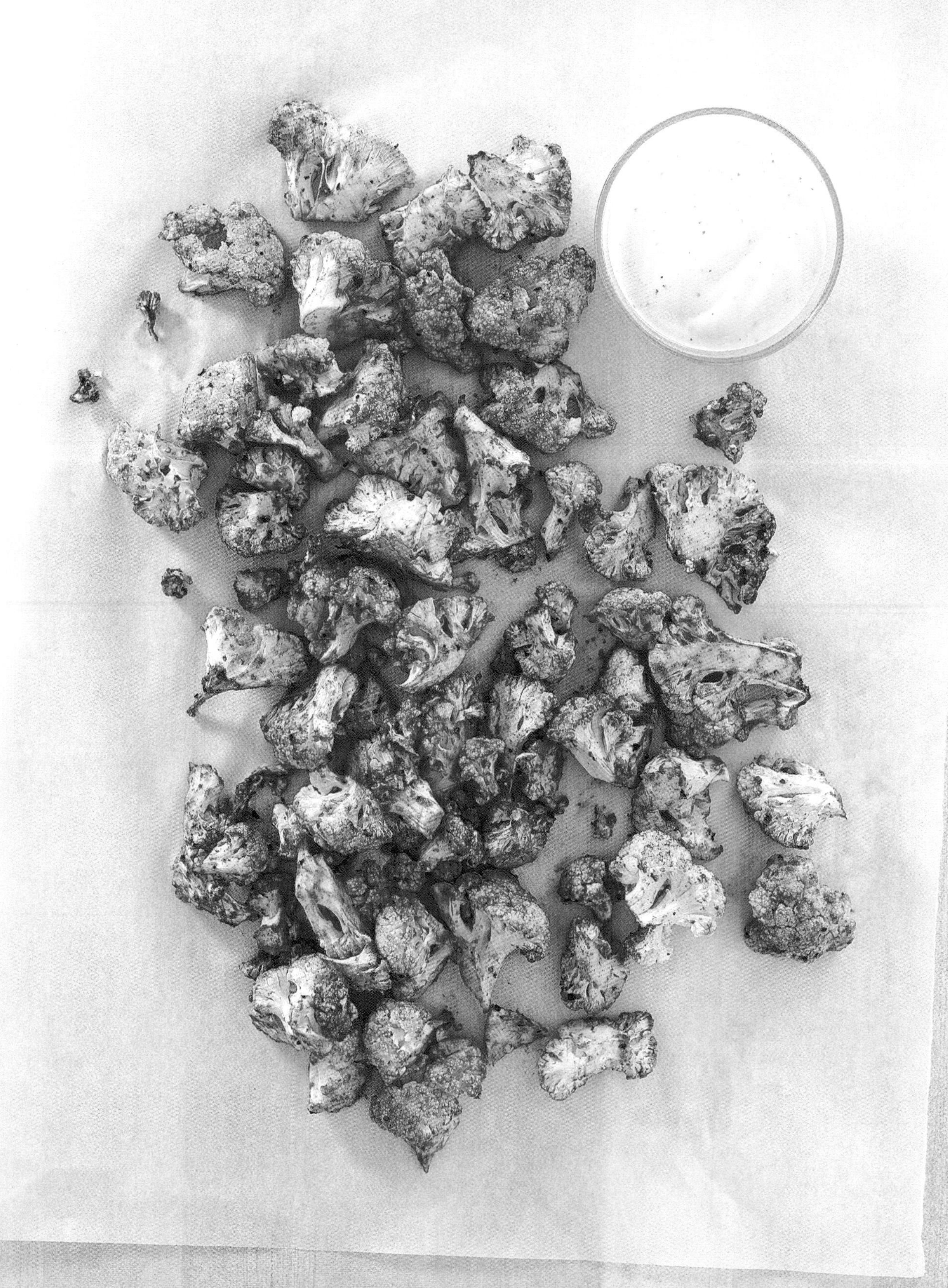

Air-Fried Buffalo Cauliflower

If you don't have an air fryer, you can make these in the oven instead. Follow the instructions as written, but instead of air frying, roast at 425°F for about 25 minutes or until cauliflower is tender and slightly crispy on the outside.

SERVES 6

Per Serving:

Calories	221
Fat	20g
Sodium	1,243mg
Carbohydrates	8g
Fiber	2g
Sugar	2g
Protein	2g

1 teaspoon garlic powder
1 teaspoon onion powder
1 teaspoon smoked paprika
1 teaspoon sea salt
½ teaspoon ground black pepper
1 large head cauliflower, cut into bite-sized florets
⅔ cup The New Primal Noble Made Medium Buffalo Sauce
¾ cup Tessemae's Creamy Ranch Dressing

1. Preheat air fryer to 375°F.
2. Combine garlic powder, onion powder, paprika, salt, and pepper in a large bowl.
3. Add cauliflower to spice mixture and toss to coat evenly. Pour buffalo sauce on top and toss again to coat.
4. Grease air fryer basket with avocado oil cooking spray. Arrange cauliflower in air fryer basket.
5. Fry for 15 minutes, turning cauliflower once while cooking. Remove from air fryer and allow to cool 30 minutes.
6. Transfer equal amounts of cauliflower into each of six airtight containers. Add 2 tablespoons ranch dressing to each of six small containers. Place small containers in large containers, cover, and store in refrigerator until ready to eat, up to 1 week.
7. When ready to serve, reheat in air fryer or under a broiler on low (watching carefully) for 2–3 minutes or until cauliflower crisps up.

REGULAR PAPRIKA VERSUS SMOKED PAPRIKA

Normal paprika is made of crushed dried chiles, whereas smoked paprika is made from chiles that have been smoke-dried and then crushed. While it seems like a minor difference, oak is used during the smoking process, and it imparts a strong woodsy flavor that has a big impact on the finished product. If you don't have smoked paprika, you won't be able to replicate the flavor exactly, but you can use regular paprika with a bit of chipotle chile powder or liquid smoke.

Samoa Energy Balls

YIELDS 12 BALLS

Per Serving (1 ball):

Calories	157
Fat	4g
Sodium	52mg
Carbohydrates	29g
Fiber	4g
Sugar	26g
Protein	1g

Adapted from the beloved Girl Scouts cookie, the Samoa, these Samoa Energy Balls don't have any added sugar, but the dates are high in natural sugar and do add a considerable amount of carbs. Because of this, they make an excellent pre-workout snack.

1 cup unsweetened shredded coconut

2 cups pitted Medjool dates

2 tablespoons Lily's stevia-sweetened chocolate chips

1 tablespoon no-sugar-added natural almond butter

¼ teaspoon sea salt

½ teaspoon vanilla extract

1. Preheat oven to 400°F. Line a baking sheet with parchment paper.
2. Spread out shredded coconut on prepared baking sheet and bake 5 minutes or until coconut starts to turn golden brown. Remove from oven.
3. Transfer ⅔ cup toasted coconut to a food processor and add remaining ingredients. Process until mixture forms a large dough ball, about 2 minutes.
4. Remove mixture from food processor and shape into twelve balls. Roll each ball in remaining toasted coconut to coat evenly.
5. Transfer balls to an airtight container and store in refrigerator up to 2 weeks or in freezer up to 3 months until ready to eat. Serve cold.

Pumpkin Oatmeal Bars

Pumpkin gets the most attention in the fall months, but these bars are the perfect snack all year round. Make sure you're buying pumpkin purée, not pumpkin pie filling. Pumpkin purée contains only pumpkin, while pumpkin pie filling contains loads of sugar (and carbs).

YIELDS 8 BARS

Per Serving (1 bar):

Calories	237
Fat	4g
Sodium	9mg
Carbohydrates	45g
Fiber	7g
Sugar	3g
Protein	7g

1 tablespoon salted grass-fed butter, melted
¼ cup Swerve brown sweetener
¼ cup Swerve granular sweetener
½ teaspoon vanilla extract
¾ cup pumpkin purée
1 teaspoon baking powder
½ teaspoon baking soda
½ teaspoon pumpkin spice powder
¼ teaspoon ground cinnamon
1½ cups gluten-free rolled oats

1. Preheat oven to 350°F. Spray an 8" × 8" baking dish with avocado oil cooking spray.
2. Combine butter and both sweeteners in a large bowl. Stir in vanilla and pumpkin purée. Add remaining ingredients and gently stir to combine.
3. Transfer mixture to prepared baking dish and spread out evenly. Bake 15 minutes or until edges are starting to turn golden brown and a toothpick inserted in center comes out clean.
4. Allow to cool 1 hour, then cut into eight bars. Transfer to individual airtight containers or reusable bags. Cover and store in refrigerator up to 1 week or in freezer up to 3 months, until ready to eat. If frozen, allow to thaw at room temperature 1 hour before eating.

Chickpea Broccoli Bites

SERVES 4

Per Serving (2 bites):

Calories	255
Fat	14g
Sodium	343mg
Carbohydrates	22g
Fiber	8g
Sugar	1g
Protein	11g

These Chickpea Broccoli Bites add some fiber and protein to any meal. They're great alongside meat, on top of salads, or with an over-easy egg.

2 cups bite-sized broccoli florets

1 (15-ounce) can chickpeas, drained and rinsed

1 large egg, lightly beaten

¼ cup almond meal

¼ cup shredded Cheddar cheese

1 teaspoon garlic powder

1 teaspoon onion powder

½ teaspoon sea salt

¼ teaspoon ground black pepper

2 tablespoons avocado oil

1. Bring a large pot of water to a boil over high heat. Add broccoli and cook until starting to soften, about 6 minutes. Add chickpeas and cook 2 minutes. Drain and transfer to a large mixing bowl.
2. Using a fork or potato masher, mash broccoli and chickpeas together. Add remaining ingredients, except oil, and mix until combined. Form mixture into eight equal balls.
3. Heat oil in a large skillet over medium-high heat. Add balls to pan and press down slightly to form patties. Cook 3 minutes, then flip and cook another 3 minutes. Remove from heat and transfer to a paper towel–lined plate. Allow to cool 10 minutes.
4. Cover and store in an airtight container in refrigerator until ready to eat, up to 1 week.
5. When ready to serve, reheat in air fryer or under a broiler on low (watching carefully) 2–3 minutes or until bites crisp up.

Paleo Meatballs

If you can't find meatloaf mix—or you want a different macro profile—you can use any combination of ground beef, pork, veal, and/or turkey. Keep in mind that the cooking times may vary a little bit depending on which meats you use.

SERVES 6

Per Serving:

Calories	337
Fat	26g
Sodium	537mg
Carbohydrates	1g
Fiber	0g
Sugar	0g
Protein	23g

⅓ cup almond meal
½ cup unsweetened almond milk
1½ pounds ground meatloaf mix
2 large eggs, lightly beaten
3 cloves garlic, peeled and minced
¼ cup chopped fresh parsley
2 tablespoons grated Parmesan cheese
1 tablespoon minced dried onion
2 teaspoons Italian seasoning
1 teaspoon salt
½ teaspoon ground black pepper

1. Preheat oven to 425°F. Line a baking sheet with parchment paper.
2. Stir almond meal and almond milk together in a small bowl. Let sit 10 minutes.
3. While almond meal is soaking, combine remaining ingredients in a large bowl. Add soaked almond meal and mix well.
4. Divide mixture into twenty-four equal balls and arrange in a single layer on prepared baking sheet. Bake 20 minutes or until meatballs are cooked through and start to turn golden brown.
5. Allow to cool 30 minutes, then transfer four meatballs to each of six airtight containers, cover, and store in refrigerator up to 1 week or in freezer up to 3 months, until ready to eat.
6. When ready to serve, arrange meatballs in a single layer on a baking sheet, cover, and cook at 300°F 10 minutes or until heated through.

Sweet Potato and Zucchini Fritters

SERVES 6

Per Serving (2 fritters):

Calories	70
Fat	3g
Sodium	425mg
Carbohydrates	6g
Fiber	1g
Sugar	1g
Protein	4g

If you want to cut down on the carbs in these fritters, you can use 2 cups of zucchini instead of a mix of sweet potato and zucchini. You can also pan-fry them if you have some room in your fat macros and want them a little crispier. Air frying is also an option. If it fits your macros, enjoy these with some no-sugar-added ketchup.

1 cup shredded zucchini
1 cup peeled shredded sweet potato
1 teaspoon salt
⅔ cup almond meal
2 large eggs, lightly beaten
1 teaspoon garlic powder
1 teaspoon onion powder
½ teaspoon ground black pepper

1. Preheat oven to 400°F. Line a baking sheet with parchment paper.
2. Combine zucchini and sweet potato in a strainer and sprinkle salt on top. Let sit 10 minutes to sweat. Transfer zucchini and sweet potatoes to a cheesecloth or nut bag and squeeze out excess liquid.
3. Put zucchini and sweet potato in a large bowl and add remaining ingredients. Mix well. Divide mixture into twelve equal portions and use your hands to form each portion into a patty or thick pancake shape.
4. Arrange fritters on prepared baking sheet and bake 20 minutes, flipping once halfway through.
5. Remove from oven and allow to cool. When ready to serve, reheat in air fryer or under a broiler on low (watching carefully) 2–3 minutes or until fritters crisp up.

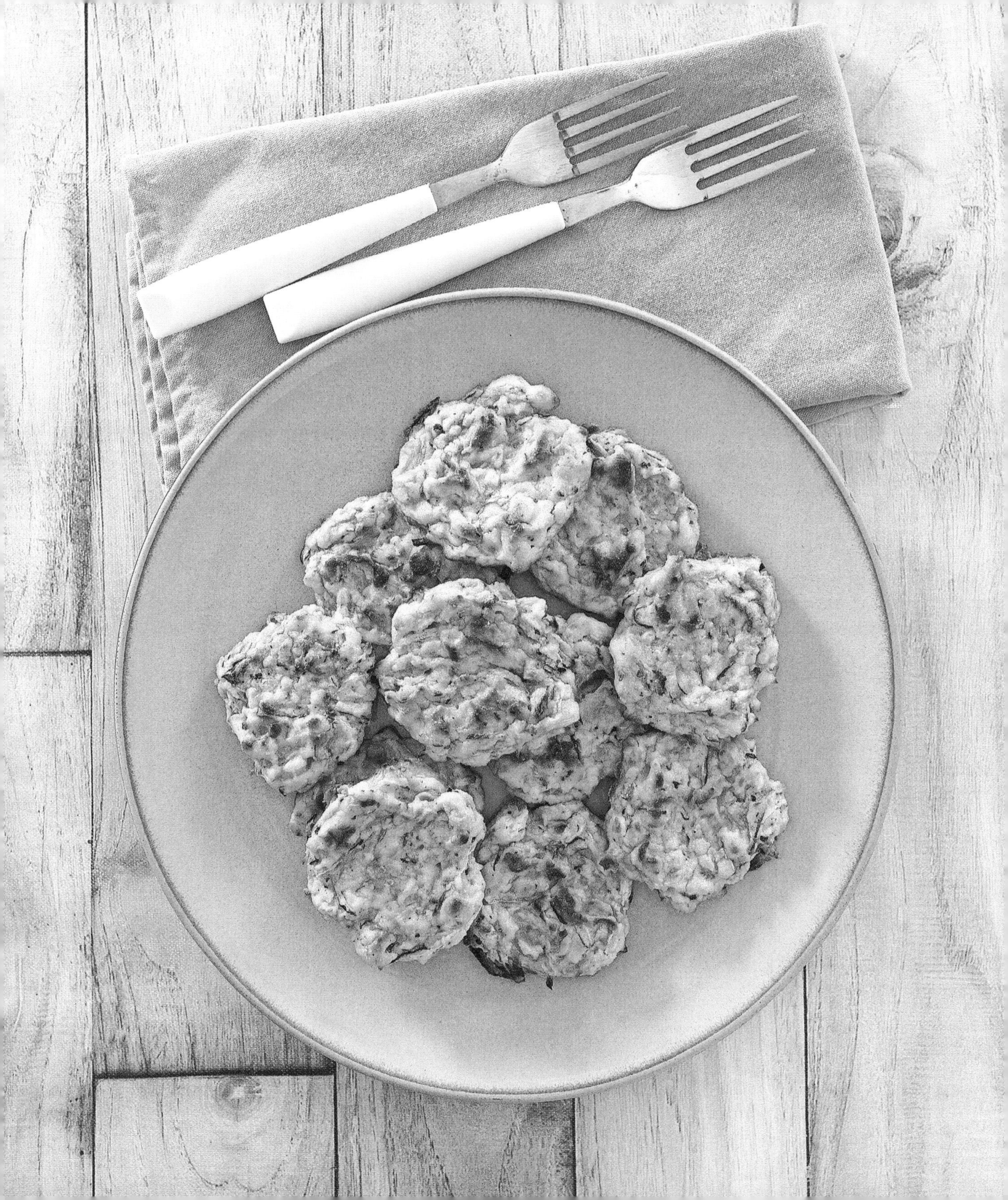

Banana Blender Muffins

YIELDS 12 MUFFINS

Per Serving (1 muffin):

Calories	133
Fat	7g
Sodium	92mg
Carbohydrates	14g
Fiber	6g
Sugar	3g
Protein	4g

FREEZE YOUR BANANAS

Next time you have a bunch of bananas that got too ripe before you could eat them, peel them, break them in half and arrange them in a single layer on a parchment paper–lined baking sheet. Freeze for 1 hour, then transfer the bananas to a freezer-safe gallon bag and store in the freezer until you're ready to use them. When ready to use the bananas, allow them to soften at room temperature for 1 hour before adding them to the blender.

These Banana Blender Muffins could not be easier. Just throw all the ingredients into a high-speed blender, then pour your batter into a muffin tin, bake, and you're done. With such little effort, they'll likely become a regular part of your meal prep rotation.

2 small ripe bananas
2 large eggs
⅓ cup unsweetened vanilla almond milk
½ cup no-sugar-added almond butter
¼ cup ChocZero Maple-Flavored Syrup
1 cup gluten-free rolled oats
1 teaspoon vanilla extract
½ teaspoon baking soda
1 teaspoon ground cinnamon
¼ teaspoon ground nutmeg
¼ teaspoon sea salt

1. Preheat oven to 350°F. Spray a twelve-cup muffin tin with avocado oil cooking spray.
2. Add all ingredients to a high-speed blender. Blend 1 minute or until smooth.
3. Pour equal amounts of batter into each muffin cup. Bake 15 minutes or until a toothpick inserted in center comes out clean.
4. Transfer muffins to an airtight container or reusable bag. Cover and store in refrigerator up to 1 week or in freezer up to 3 months, until ready to eat.
5. Allow to come to room temperature before serving.

Protein Cauliflower Tots

The chickpea flour in these Protein Cauliflower Tots not only helps hold everything together, but it also adds some extra protein to help fill you up. If you don't have it, it's worth adding to your macro-friendly pantry.

SERVES 4

Per Serving:

Calories	106
Fat	2g
Sodium	640mg
Carbohydrates	15g
Fiber	3g
Sugar	3g
Protein	7g

3 cups cauliflower florets
¾ cup chickpea flour
1 large egg, lightly beaten
1 teaspoon garlic powder
1 teaspoon sea salt
½ teaspoon dried minced onion
½ teaspoon smoked paprika
¼ teaspoon ground black pepper

1. Preheat oven to 425°F. Line a baking sheet with parchment paper.
2. Bring a large pot of water to a boil over high heat. Add cauliflower and cook 8 minutes or until cauliflower is extra tender. Drain and transfer cauliflower to a food processor or high-speed blender. Process 2 minutes or until smooth.
3. Transfer cauliflower to a cheesecloth or nut bag and squeeze out excess liquid. Put cauliflower in a large mixing bowl, add remaining ingredients, and mix well.
4. Scoop mixture out into tablespoonfuls and shape into tots. Arrange in a single layer on prepared baking sheet.
5. Bake 20 minutes, turning tots over halfway through cooking. Remove from oven and allow to cool 30 minutes.
6. Divide tots evenly into four airtight containers. Cover and store in refrigerator up to 1 week or in freezer up to 3 months, until ready to eat.
7. When ready to serve, reheat in air fryer or under a broiler on low (watching carefully) 2–3 minutes or until tots crisp up.

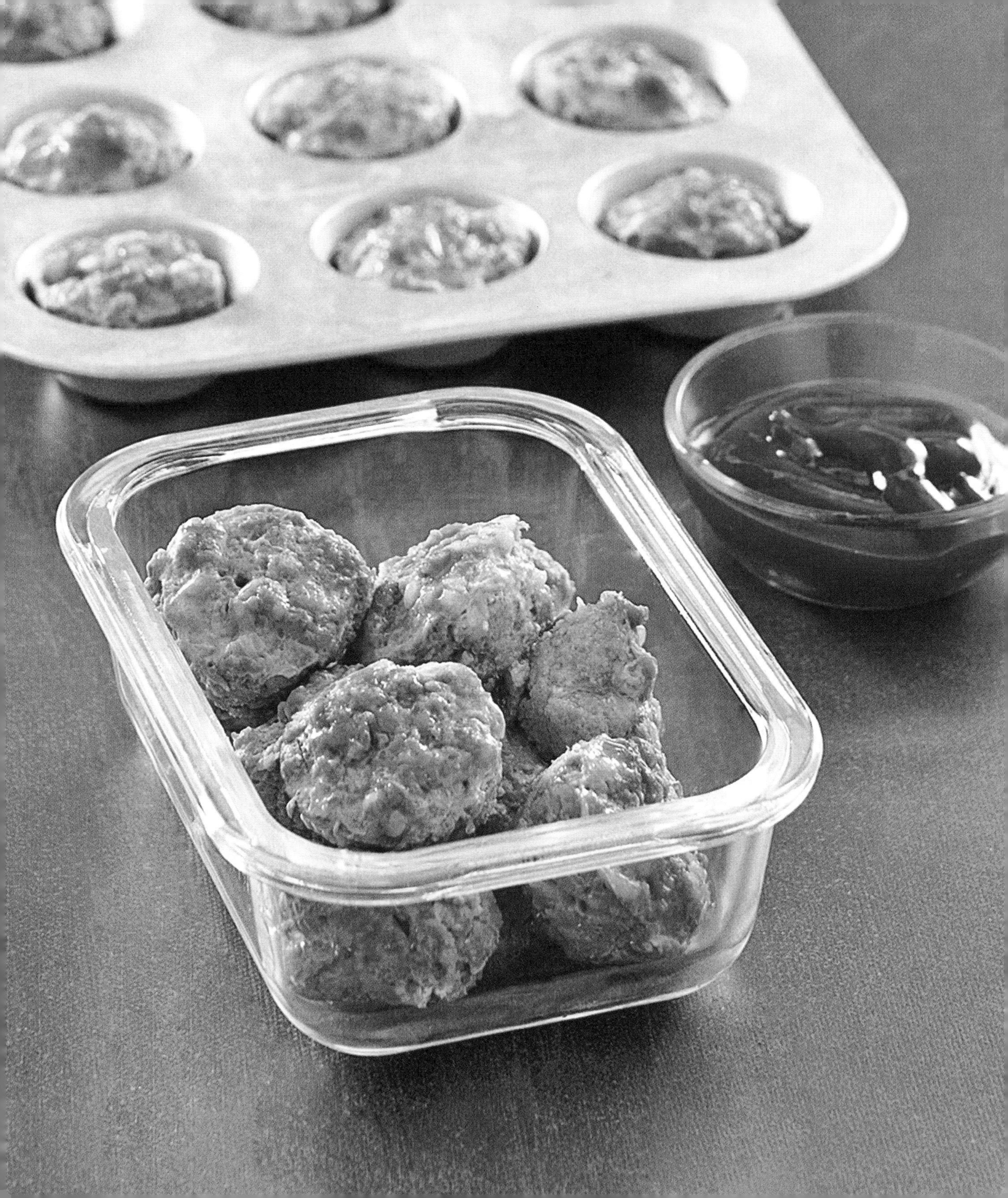

Crispy Cheeseburger Bites

These Crispy Cheeseburger Bites are a great snack to help hold you over until your next meal, and if it fits your macros they pair well with no-sugar-added ketchup as a dip. They also make an easy, portable source of protein to add to salads or any other meals.

SERVES 12

Per Serving:

Calories	110
Fat	7g
Sodium	207mg
Carbohydrates	1g
Fiber	0g
Sugar	1g
Protein	10g

¼ cup almond meal

2 tablespoons unsweetened almond milk

1 pound 90% lean ground turkey

4 large egg whites

½ cup shredded Cheddar cheese

½ cup shredded Parmesan cheese

¼ cup Tessemae's Unsweetened Ketchup

3 tablespoons yellow mustard

3 small dill pickles, finely diced

1. Preheat oven to 400°F. Spray a twenty-four-cup mini muffin tin with avocado oil cooking spray.
2. Combine almond meal and almond milk in a small bowl and let sit 10 minutes.
3. While almond meal is soaking, combine remaining ingredients in a large bowl. Add soaked almond meal and mix well.
4. Divide mixture into twenty-four equal balls and press into each muffin cup.
5. Bake 30 minutes or until turkey is cooked through. Remove from oven and allow to cool 30 minutes.
6. Transfer two bites to each of twelve airtight containers or reusable bags. Cover and store in refrigerator up to 1 week or until ready to eat.
7. When ready to serve, reheat in air fryer or under a broiler on low (watching carefully) 2–3 minutes or until bites crisp up.

CHAPTER 11

Sweets and Treats

Cookies and Cream Protein Cheesecake

SERVES 9

Per Serving:

Calories	271
Fat	23g
Sodium	255mg
Carbohydrates	5g
Fiber	0g
Sugar	3g
Protein	12g

For this recipe you can use any cookies and cream protein that fits into your macros. However, keep in mind that some are loaded with artificial ingredients that may not add carbohydrates or fat, but they also don't promote optimal health.

FOR CRUST

1 cup almond flour

¼ cup Swerve granular sweetener

2 tablespoons unsalted grass-fed butter, melted

FOR FILLING

16 ounces cream cheese, softened

1 cup 2% plain Greek yogurt

¼ cup Legion Whey+ Cookies and Cream Whey Protein Powder

1 large egg

2 large egg whites

1½ teaspoons vanilla extract

¼ cup Swerve granular sweetener

⅛ teaspoon sea salt

1. To make Crust: Preheat oven to 350°F. Line a 9" springform pan with parchment paper.
2. Combine almond flour and sweetener in a small bowl. Add butter and mix until crumbly mixture forms. Press into prepared pan in an even layer.
3. Bake 8 minutes or until crust starts to turn slightly golden brown.
4. To make Filling: While crust is baking, add cream cheese and yogurt to a stand mixer (or use an electric hand mixer and a mixing bowl) and beat 1 minute or until light and fluffy. Beat in protein powder, egg, egg whites, and vanilla. Add sweetener and salt and lightly beat just until incorporated.
5. Pour mixture over prepared Crust and spread out evenly with a spatula.
6. Bake 30 minutes, then decrease oven temperature to 200°F (without opening oven door) and bake 50–60 minutes until cheesecake is set.
7. Remove from oven and allow to cool completely, about 1 hour. Transfer to refrigerator, cover, and allow to chill overnight.
8. Remove rim of springform pan and cut cheesecake into nine slices. Transfer each slice to a separate airtight container, cover, and store in refrigerator up to 1 week, until ready to eat.

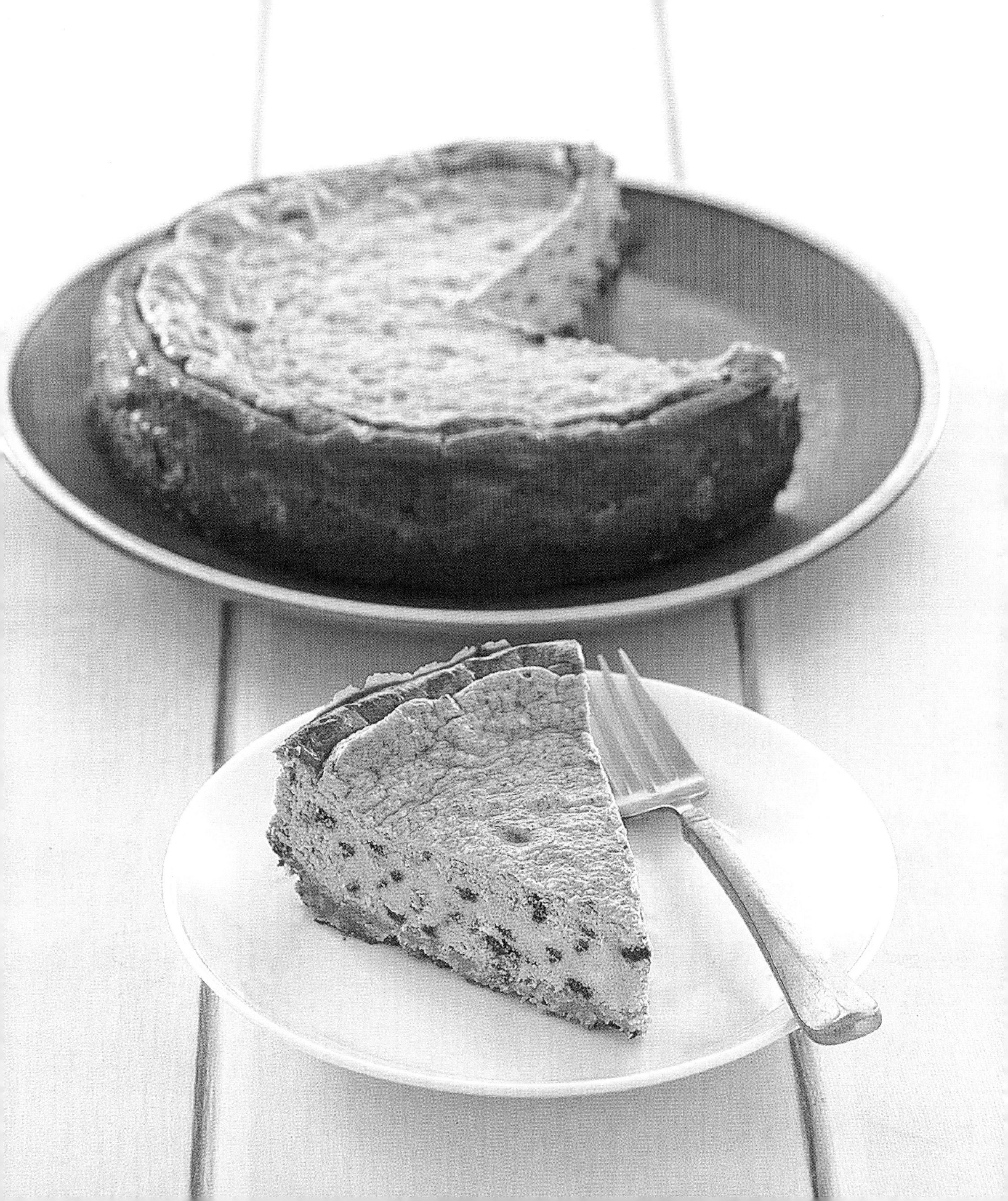

Carrot Cake Bites

YIELDS 12 BITES

Per Serving (1 bite):

Calories	114
Fat	2g
Sodium	70mg
Carbohydrates	16g
Fiber	3g
Sugar	13g
Protein	8g

If these Carrot Cake Bites have a bit too many carbs for your liking, you can cut the dates down to 3⁄4 or 2⁄3 cup. That's enough to help them stick together, but it will lower the sugar content considerably.

1 cup pitted Medjool dates
½ cup crushed walnuts
½ cup Tera's Whey vanilla protein powder
2 tablespoons unsweetened vanilla almond milk
1 teaspoon ground cinnamon
⅛ teaspoon ground allspice
⅛ teaspoon ground nutmeg
⅛ teaspoon sea salt
1 cup peeled shredded carrots

1. Line an 8" × 8" baking dish with parchment paper.
2. Add dates to a food processor and pulse 30 seconds. Add remaining ingredients, except carrots, and process until smooth, about 2 minutes. Add carrots and pulse until incorporated but not fully blended, about 30 seconds.
3. Transfer mixture to prepared baking dish and press down evenly. Freeze 20 minutes or until set.
4. Cut into twelve bars and transfer to an airtight container. Store in freezer until ready to eat, up to 3 months. Allow to come to room temperature before serving.

No-Bake Peanut Butter Protein Cookies

If you can't have peanut butter, or prefer not to, you can use any type of nut or seed butter in its place. Just make sure it isn't too runny, or the cookies won't hold their shape well.

YIELDS 12 COOKIES

Per Serving (1 cookie):

Calories	246
Fat	11g
Sodium	35mg
Carbohydrates	25g
Fiber	5g
Sugar	1g
Protein	12g

1 cup no-sugar-added chunky peanut butter

2 tablespoons ChocZero Maple-Flavored Syrup

1 tablespoon unsweetened almond milk

¼ cup Tera's Whey vanilla protein powder

1½ cups gluten-free rolled oats

⅛ teaspoon sea salt

1. Line a baking sheet with parchment paper.
2. Combine peanut butter, maple syrup, and almond milk in a large bowl. Add remaining ingredients and mix until a dough forms.
3. Divide mixture into twelve equal portions, roll into balls, and place in a single layer on prepared baking sheet. Flatten balls slightly to resemble cookies. Refrigerate 1 hour until set.
4. Transfer to an airtight container, cover, and store in refrigerator up to 1 week or in freezer up to 3 months, until ready to eat. Allow to come to room temperature before serving.

ROLLED OATS VERSUS INSTANT OATS

Rolled oats, often called old-fashioned oats, are oats that have been steamed and flattened into flakes. They cook more quickly than steel-cut oats but not as fast as quick-cooking or instant oats. In recipes that don't require any cooking, you can use rolled oats and instant oats interchangeably, but if you need to cook your recipe, you'll have to adjust the cooking time to compensate.

Chocolate Chip Oatmeal Balls

YIELDS 8 BALLS

Per Serving (1 ball):

Calories	170
Fat	7g
Sodium	46mg
Carbohydrates	17g
Fiber	3g
Sugar	3g
Protein	10g

The honey in this recipe is vital for helping everything stick together, so you can't replace it with Swerve granular sweetener. If you don't want the extra carbs, you can use one of the ChocZero low-carb syrups in its place.

¾ cup gluten-free rolled oats
¼ cup Tera's Whey vanilla protein powder
¼ cup no-sugar-added sunflower seed butter
1 tablespoon raw honey
½ teaspoon vanilla extract
3 tablespoons Lily's stevia-sweetened chocolate chips

1. Line a baking sheet with parchment paper.
2. Mix together oats and protein powder in a large bowl. Add sunflower seed butter, honey, and vanilla and mix to combine. Fold in chocolate chips.
3. Divide mixture into eight equal portions. Roll each portion into a ball and place on prepared baking sheet. Chill in refrigerator 3 hours.
4. Transfer balls to an airtight container, cover, and store in refrigerator until ready to eat, up to 1 week.

WHY WHEY?

Whey protein is not only a complete protein but is also highly bioavailable and easy to digest, meaning that your body is absorbing the protein and amino acids you're consuming. If you prefer not to use whey, you can swap it out for your favorite plant-based protein powder, but you'll lose some of the essential amino acids in the process. Whichever protein you choose, make sure to diligently read labels so you'll land on one that's free of added sugar and artificial ingredients.

Cinnamon Almond Butter Protein Balls

These Cinnamon Almond Butter Protein Balls are an excellent way to get in a healthy dose of protein when you're on the go or in between meals. You can keep a couple with you and eat them as a pre- or post-workout snack.

YIELDS 8 BALLS

Per Serving (1 ball):

Calories	149
Fat	4g
Sodium	31mg
Carbohydrates	18g
Fiber	3g
Sugar	3g
Protein	10g

3⁄4 cup gluten-free rolled oats

1⁄4 cup Tera's Whey vanilla protein powder

1⁄4 cup no-sugar-added almond butter

1 tablespoon raw honey

1⁄4 teaspoon almond extract

2 tablespoons crushed almonds

1. Line a baking sheet with parchment paper.
2. Mix together oats and protein powder in a large bowl. Add almond butter, honey, and almond extract and mix to combine. Fold in crushed almonds.
3. Divide mixture into eight equal portions. Roll each portion into a ball and place on prepared baking sheet. Chill in refrigerator 3 hours.
4. Transfer balls to an airtight container and store in refrigerator until ready to eat, up to 1 week.

Strawberries with Chocolate Cheesecake Dip

SERVES 6

Per Serving:	
Calories	126
Fat	6g
Sodium	90mg
Carbohydrates	15g
Fiber	3g
Sugar	10g
Protein	3g

This recipe can be easily customized to fit into your macros. If you have room for more carbs, you can use regular TruWhip rather than the keto version. If you can spare some fat grams, you can play around with the fat percentage of the yogurt and/or cream cheese.

¾ cup TruWhip keto whipped topping
⅓ cup 2% plain Greek yogurt
¼ cup softened cream cheese
2 tablespoons unsweetened cocoa powder
2 tablespoons Swerve granular sweetener
1 teaspoon vanilla extract
⅛ teaspoon sea salt
6 cups whole strawberries

1. Add all ingredients, except strawberries, to a food processor or large mixing bowl. Process until smooth.
2. Transfer equal amounts of dip to each of six airtight containers. Add 1 cup strawberries to each container. Cover and refrigerate until ready to eat, up to 1 week.

Strawberry Shortcake Chia Pudding

SERVES 6

Per Serving:	
Calories	117
Fat	3g
Sodium	413mg
Carbohydrates	14g
Fiber	9g
Sugar	3g
Protein	8g

This chia pudding is loaded with protein thanks to the Greek yogurt and collagen powder. You can eat it for a sweet treat or have it for breakfast and stay full all morning.

3 cups unsweetened vanilla almond milk
¼ cup 2% plain Greek yogurt
¼ cup chia seeds
2 scoops Vital Proteins Collagen Peptides
2 tablespoons ChocZero Maple-Flavored Syrup
2 tablespoons vanilla extract
¾ teaspoon sea salt
1½ cups chopped frozen strawberries

1. Add all ingredients, except strawberries, to a blender. Blend 30 seconds until smooth.
2. Pour mixture evenly into six pint-sized Mason jars. Add ¼ cup chopped strawberries to each jar. Cover and shake vigorously.
3. Refrigerate 4 hours until set. Store in refrigerator until ready to eat, up to 1 week.

S'more Protein Bites

Dandies marshmallows contain sugar, but they're a better-for-you option than the typical marshmallows you'll find in grocery stores. If you can't find them, you can use any type of marshmallow in their place, but keep in mind that the swap will change the macros slightly.

YIELDS 12 BITES

Per Serving (1 bite):

Calories	137
Fat	4g
Sodium	30mg
Carbohydrates	19g
Fiber	6g
Sugar	3g
Protein	7g

1 cup gluten-free rolled oats
⅓ cup crushed gluten-free graham crackers
1 tablespoon chia seeds
¼ cup Tera's Whey vanilla protein powder
¼ cup unsweetened vanilla almond milk
2 tablespoons ChocZero Maple-Flavored Syrup
¼ cup Lily's stevia-sweetened chocolate chips
¼ cup chopped Dandies marshmallows

1. Combine oats, graham crackers, chia seeds, and protein powder in a large bowl. Add almond milk and maple syrup and stir until a dough forms.
2. Mix in chocolate chips and marshmallow pieces, then divide mixture into twelve equal portions and roll into balls.
3. Transfer to an airtight container, cover, and store in refrigerator until ready to eat, up to 2 weeks.

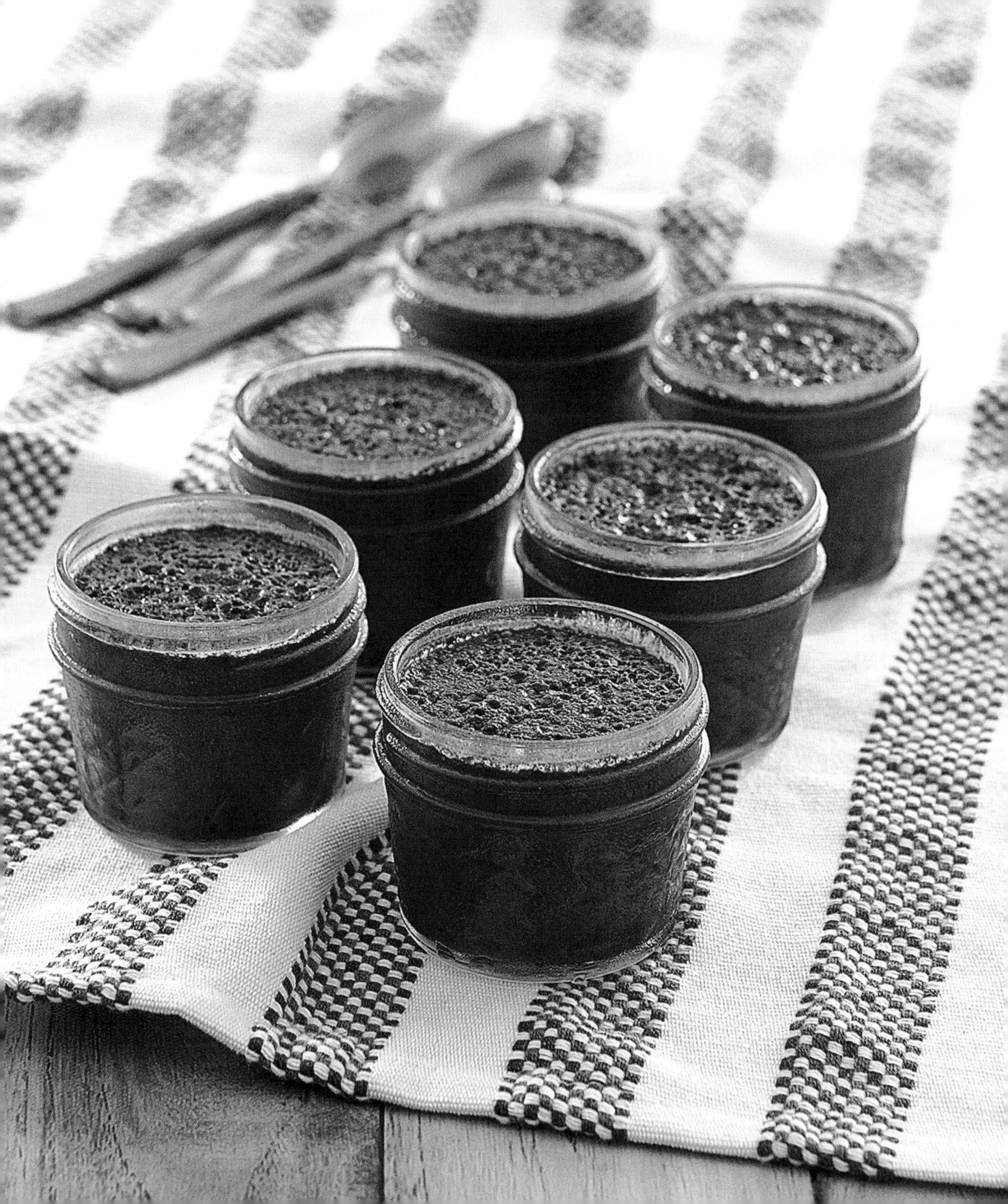

Chocolate Chia Seed Pudding

The longer this chia seed pudding sits in the refrigerator, the thicker it will get. If you don't like it extra thick, you can stir in a little more almond milk before eating it to get it to your desired consistency. Just make sure to account for this when tracking your macros.

SERVES 6

Per Serving:

Calories	109
Fat	5g
Sodium	109mg
Carbohydrates	7g
Fiber	5g
Sugar	1g
Protein	9g

3 cups unsweetened almond milk

¼ cup Tera's Whey chocolate protein powder

5 tablespoons chia seeds

1. Add all ingredients to a shaker cup or large airtight container. Shake vigorously 30 seconds.
2. Pour equal portions into each of six pint-sized Mason jars or other airtight containers and cover.
3. Refrigerate at least 4 hours until set. Store in refrigerator until ready to eat, up to 1 week.

Double Chocolate Fudge Bites

YIELDS 12 BITES

Per Serving (1 bite):

Calories	134
Fat	7g
Sodium	69mg
Carbohydrates	11g
Fiber	10g
Sugar	0g
Protein	7g

THE POWER OF CHIA SEEDS

Chia seeds are a great tool for baking because they absorb water and expand, acting as a thickener and a stabilizer. They're also a great way to add extra fiber and protein to baked goods that are otherwise lacking in micronutrients. Chia seeds can also be used to replace eggs in baking, helping turn baked goods into a vegan-friendly treat. For each egg you want to replace, mix 1 tablespoon chia seeds with 3 tablespoons water in a small bowl. Wait 5 minutes or until a gel forms, and then use it in your recipe as you would an egg.

If you want to make this recipe vegan, simply swap out the whey protein powder for any vegan-friendly protein powder of your choice. Just make sure you check the ingredients and calculate the difference in macros to make sure it fits into your plan.

¼ cup Tera's Whey chocolate protein powder

¼ cup coconut flour

3 tablespoons unsweetened cocoa powder

2 tablespoons chia seeds

½ cup no-sugar-added sunflower seed butter

⅓ cup ChocZero Maple-Flavored Syrup

½ teaspoon vanilla extract

3 tablespoons Lily's stevia-sweetened chocolate chips

1. Line a baking sheet with parchment paper.
2. Combine protein powder, coconut flour, cocoa powder, and chia seeds in a large bowl. Stir in sunflower seed butter, maple syrup, and vanilla. Fold in chocolate chips.
3. Divide into twelve equal portions and roll into balls. Arrange in a single layer on prepared baking sheet.
4. Freeze 1 hour, then transfer to an airtight container. Cover and store in refrigerator up to 2 weeks or in freezer up to 3 months, until ready to eat. Allow to come to room temperature before serving.

Edible Protein Cookie Dough

The cookie dough is arguably the best part of making cookies. This high-protein (and raw egg-free) cookie dough makes a great dessert right out of the container with a spoon, or you can eat it with gluten-free graham crackers if you have some carb macros to spare.

SERVES 12

Per Serving:

Calories	86
Fat	4g
Sodium	51mg
Carbohydrates	9g
Fiber	4g
Sugar	0g
Protein	3g

1 (15-ounce) can chickpeas, drained and rinsed

¼ teaspoon sea salt

⅛ teaspoon baking soda

1 teaspoon vanilla extract

¼ cup no-sugar-added cashew butter

2 tablespoons unsweetened almond milk

3 tablespoons Swerve granular sweetener

2 tablespoons ground flaxseeds

⅓ cup Lily's stevia-sweetened chocolate chips

1. Add all ingredients, except chocolate chips, to a food processor. Process 2 minutes until smooth.
2. Stir in chocolate chips.
3. Divide cookie dough evenly into twelve airtight containers. Store in refrigerator up to 2 weeks or in freezer up to 3 months, until ready to eat.

Protein Buckeyes

YIELDS 16 BUCKEYES

Per Serving (2 buckeyes):

Calories	252
Fat	20g
Sodium	14mg
Carbohydrates	8g
Fiber	4g
Sugar	2g
Protein	10g

MAKING YOUR OWN CONFECTIONERS' SUGAR

Confectioners' sugar, or powdered sugar, is just a blended version of regular granulated sugar. If you only have granular Swerve, you can usually substitute it for confectioners' Swerve, or you can make your own powdered sugar in the food processor or a high-speed blender. Just add the granular sweetener and blend or process until a fine powder forms.

If these Protein Buckeyes have too much fat for your macro allowance, you can cut back on the butter slightly—¼ cup will still work.

⅔ cup no-sugar-added creamy peanut butter
⅓ cup unsalted grass-fed butter, softened
1 teaspoon vanilla extract
1 teaspoon unsweetened vanilla almond milk
¼ cup Tera's Whey protein powder
¼ cup Swerve confectioners' sweetener
½ cup Lily's stevia-sweetened chocolate chips

1. Line a baking sheet with parchment paper.
2. Add peanut butter, butter, vanilla, and almond milk to a food processor. Process 20 seconds or until smooth.
3. Add protein powder and sweetener and process until incorporated, about 30 seconds.
4. Divide mixture into sixteen equal portions. Roll into balls and arrange in a single layer on prepared baking sheet. Transfer to freezer for 20 minutes.
5. While balls are chilling, put chocolate chips in a small microwave-safe bowl. Microwave on medium heat 2 minutes, stirring every 15 seconds, or until chocolate is melted and smooth. Set aside to cool slightly.
6. Remove peanut butter balls from freezer. Using a toothpick or fork, dip each ball halfway into chocolate and then return to baking sheet. Repeat until all balls are coated. Return to freezer for 20 minutes or until chocolate is set.
7. Transfer balls to an airtight container, cover, and store in refrigerator up to 1 week or in freezer up to 3 months, until ready to eat.

Paleo Apple Pie Bars

Check your ingredient labels and make sure the applesauce you use in this recipe has no added sugar. Sweetened applesauce contains about 43 grams per cup, while unsweetened applesauce has 27 grams, all from apples.

2 tablespoons apple butter
2 tablespoons no-sugar-added almond butter
½ cup ChocZero Maple-Flavored Syrup
½ cup unsweetened applesauce
3 tablespoons unsweetened vanilla almond milk
1 cup coconut flour
½ cup almond flour
½ cup Tera's Whey vanilla protein powder
2 tablespoons Swerve granular sweetener
2 teaspoons ground cinnamon
1 teaspoon ground allspice
½ teaspoon ground nutmeg

1. Line a 9" × 9" baking dish with parchment paper.
2. Add apple butter, almond butter, and maple syrup to a large mixing bowl. Use a handheld or stand mixer to mix until smooth, about 30 seconds. Add applesauce and almond milk and mix 15 seconds.
3. Add remaining ingredients and mix until smooth, another 30 seconds.
4. Transfer mixture to prepared baking dish and press to spread evenly. Refrigerate 1 hour until set.
5. Lift parchment paper out of baking dish and cut mixture into twelve bars. Transfer bars to an airtight container, cover, and store in refrigerator up to 2 weeks or in freezer up to 3 months.

YIELDS 12 BARS

Per Serving (1 bar):

Calories	132
Fat	4g
Sodium	50mg
Carbohydrates	15g
Fiber	13g
Sugar	3g
Protein	9g

MAKING YOUR OWN APPLE BUTTER

Apple butter is simple to make. Combine 3 pounds apples (peeled, cored, and sliced) with ½ cup granular Swerve, ½ cup brown Swerve, 2 teaspoons ground cinnamon, ¼ teaspoon ground nutmeg, ⅛ teaspoon ground cloves, ⅛ teaspoon sea salt, and 2 teaspoons vanilla extract in a slow cooker, cover, and cook on low for 10–12 hours or until apples are broken down and smooth. Then purée with an immersion blender. Transfer to an airtight container and store in the refrigerator up to 1 week or the freezer up to 3 months.

Chocolate PB Chia Pudding

SERVES 6

Per Serving:

Calories	193
Fat	10g
Sodium	173mg
Carbohydrates	10g
Fiber	7g
Sugar	3g
Protein	16g

WHAT IS PEANUT BUTTER POWDER?

Peanut butter powder is made from peanuts that have been roasted and pressed to remove excess oil, then ground into a fine powder. Because the oil is removed, peanut butter powder is significantly lower in fat than peanut butter. For comparison, 1 tablespoon peanut butter has 8 grams of fat and 4 grams of protein, while 1 tablespoon peanut butter powder has 0.75 grams of fat and 3 grams of protein.

This Chocolate PB Chia Pudding is so simple and so delicious that it will no doubt become a staple in your meal prep routine. The peanut butter powder adds a delicious nutty flavor for considerably fewer grams of fat than regular peanut butter.

3 cups unsweetened almond milk

¼ cup Tera's Whey chocolate protein powder

5 tablespoons chia seeds

6 tablespoons peanut butter powder

6 tablespoons crushed peanuts

1. Add all ingredients to a shaker cup or other large airtight container. Shake vigorously 30 seconds.
2. Pour equal portions into each of six pint-sized Mason jars or other airtight containers and cover.
3. Refrigerate 4 hours. Store in refrigerator until ready to eat, up to 1 week.

Protein Brownie Bites

The black beans in this recipe add a hefty dose of protein and fiber—two nutrients that help keep you full, and your blood sugar steady, for hours—but thanks to the cacao powder, you won't even taste them.

YIELDS 12 BITES

Per Serving (1 bite):

Calories	162
Fat	6g
Sodium	203mg
Carbohydrates	24g
Fiber	14g
Sugar	1g
Protein	4g

1 (15-ounce) can black beans, drained and rinsed

½ cup gluten-free rolled oats

½ cup ChocZero Maple-Flavored Syrup

¼ cup Nutiva Buttery Flavor Coconut Oil

2 tablespoons raw cacao powder

1 teaspoon vanilla extract

½ teaspoon baking powder

¼ teaspoon sea salt

½ cup Lily's stevia-sweetened chocolate chips

1. Preheat oven to 350°F. Line a 12-cup muffin tin with paper or silicone liners.
2. Add all ingredients, except chocolate chips, to a food processor and process 2 minutes or until smooth.
3. Stir in chocolate chips.
4. Divide batter equally into each muffin cup. Bake 15 minutes or until brownies are cooked through. Remove from oven and allow to cool completely, about 1 hour.
5. Transfer to an airtight container, cover, and store in refrigerator until ready to eat, up to 2 weeks.

Chocolate-Covered Strawberry Protein Pops

SERVES 10

Per Serving:

Calories	95
Fat	1g
Sodium	47mg
Carbohydrates	12g
Fiber	7g
Sugar	3g
Protein	10g

If you've ever had chocolate-covered strawberries, you already know they make a great combination, but you can use any of your favorite berries in this recipe. If you want more variety in your weekly dessert, you can even make two flavors at once by dividing the mixture into two portions before blending in the berries.

1 large banana

¾ cup 2% plain Greek yogurt

1 cup unsweetened vanilla almond milk

½ teaspoon vanilla extract

¼ cup ChocZero Chocolate-Flavored Syrup

½ cup Tera's Whey chocolate protein powder

⅔ cup finely diced frozen strawberries

1. Add all ingredients, except strawberries, to a blender and blend 30 seconds or until smooth. Add strawberries and pulse 2 or 3 times to incorporate.
2. Pour equal amounts of mixture into each well of a ten-well ice pop mold. Freeze at least 2 hours until frozen. Store in freezer until ready to eat, up to 3 months.

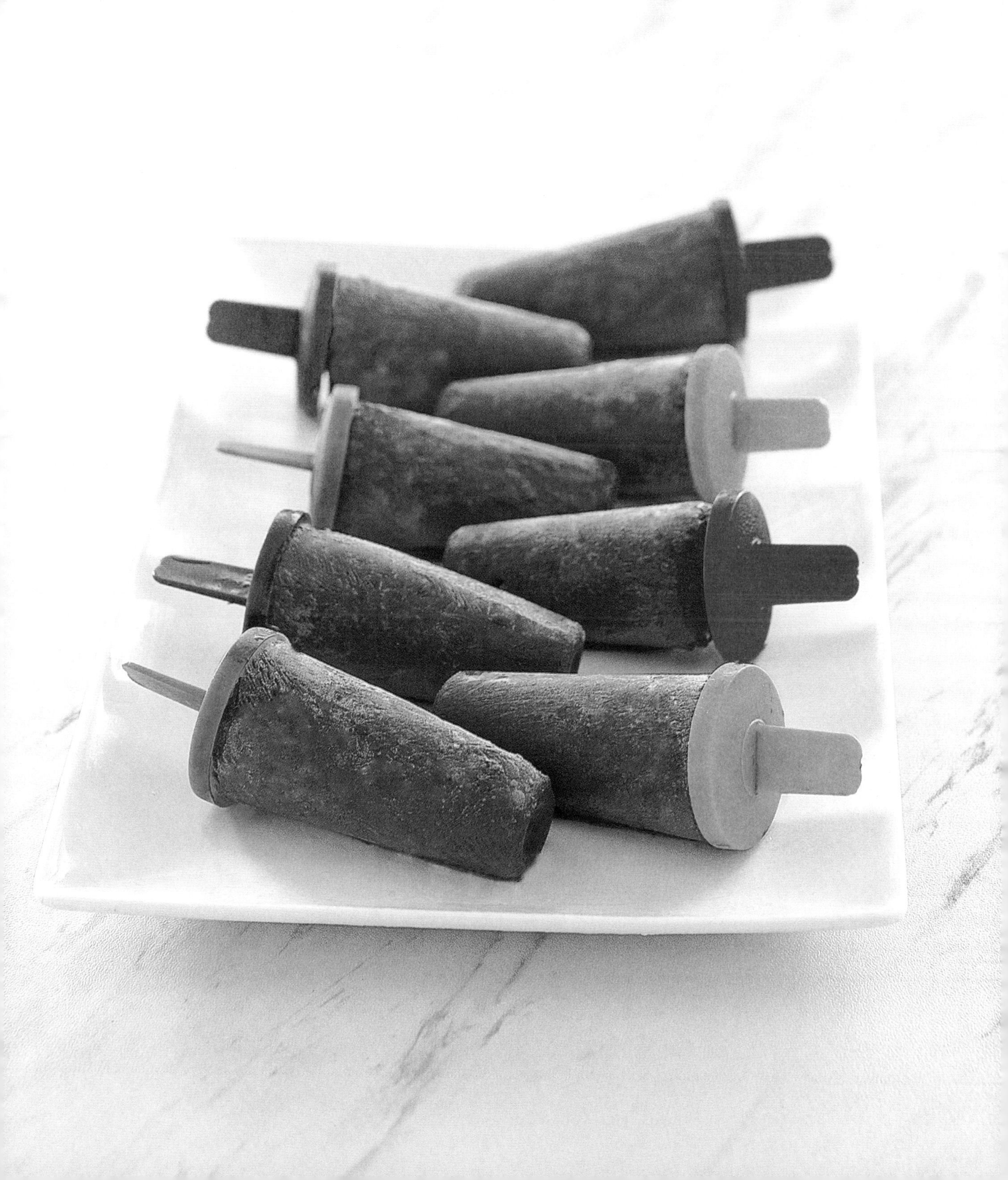

Dark Chocolate Protein Popcorn

SERVES 4

Per Serving:

Calories	164
Fat	15g
Sodium	160mg
Carbohydrates	2g
Fiber	0g
Sugar	2g
Protein	5g

When storing this popcorn, make sure you keep it in a fairly cool place. If it's too hot in your home, the coconut oil will melt—coconut oil melts at 76°F—and you'll end up with a mess. A delicious mess, but a mess nonetheless.

4 tablespoons melted Nutiva Buttery Flavor Coconut Oil, divided

½ cup organic popcorn kernels

2 tablespoons Tera's Whey chocolate protein powder

1 teaspoon unsweetened cocoa powder

1 teaspoon Swerve confectioners' sweetener

¼ teaspoon sea salt

1. Heat 1 tablespoon oil in a large saucepan over medium heat. Add a handful of kernels to oil. Once kernels begin to pop, about 5 minutes, add remaining kernels. Cover saucepan and shake to coat kernels with oil.
2. As kernels begin to pop, shake pan every few seconds to move kernels around and prevent popped corn from burning. When popping slows down to 2 seconds between pops, remove from heat and transfer popcorn to a large container.
3. Combine remaining 3 tablespoons oil, protein powder, cocoa powder, sweetener, and salt in a small bowl. Drizzle over popcorn and shake to coat.
4. Divide popcorn into four airtight containers and store at room temperature until ready to eat, up to 1 week.

Chocolate-Covered Banana Bites

Technically these bites aren't covered in chocolate, but they give you all the delicious flavors of a chocolate-covered banana in an easy-to-grab treat. You can store them in the refrigerator, but they're great right out of the freezer—and they'll last longer.

YIELDS 12 BITES

Per Serving (2 bites):

Calories	73
Fat	2g
Sodium	0mg
Carbohydrates	12g
Fiber	4g
Sugar	3g
Protein	2g

2 medium ripe bananas

1 cup gluten-free rolled oats

1 teaspoon ground cinnamon

3⁄4 teaspoon vanilla extract

3⁄4 cup Lily's stevia-sweetened chocolate chips

1. Preheat oven to 350°F. Line a baking sheet with parchment paper.
2. Add bananas to a large mixing bowl and mash with a fork. Stir in oats, cinnamon, and vanilla. Fold in chocolate chips.
3. Scoop tablespoons of mixture onto prepared baking sheet and form into twelve balls. Bake 20 minutes or until bites are set. Remove from oven and allow to cool 1 hour.
4. Transfer two bites to each of six airtight containers or reusable bags. Cover and store in refrigerator up to 1 week or in freezer up to 3 months, until ready to eat.

Fudgy Chickpea Brownies

YIELDS 12 BROWNIES

Per Serving (1 brownie):

Calories	98
Fat	4g
Sodium	53mg
Carbohydrates	13g
Fiber	12g
Sugar	0g
Protein	3g

These brownies are so fudgy, you'd never know there were chickpeas hidden inside if it weren't for the impressive protein count. Make sure they're completely cool before cutting, though, or they'll fall apart.

1 (15-ounce) can chickpeas, drained and rinsed
½ cup no-sugar-added almond butter
½ cup ChocZero Chocolate-Flavored Syrup
1 tablespoon unsweetened chocolate almond milk
1 tablespoon unsalted grass-fed butter, melted
1 teaspoon vanilla extract
¼ cup almond flour
¼ cup unsweetened cocoa powder
¼ teaspoon baking powder
¼ teaspoon baking soda
¼ teaspoon sea salt

1. Preheat oven to 350°F. Line an 8" × 8" baking dish with parchment paper.
2. Add chickpeas, almond butter, chocolate syrup, almond milk, butter, and vanilla to a food processor. Process until chickpeas are broken down and mixture is smooth, about 45 seconds. Add remaining ingredients and process 30 seconds until fully incorporated.
3. Transfer batter to prepared baking dish and use a spatula to spread evenly. Bake 20 minutes or until brownies are set. Allow to cool 1 hour.
4. Lift parchment paper out of baking dish and cut brownies into twelve squares. Transfer to an airtight container, cover, and store in refrigerator up to 1 week or in freezer up to 3 months, until ready to eat.

WHIP IT UP

If you want to take these brownies up a notch, make some aquafaba, or chickpea whipped cream, to go with it. Rather than draining the chickpeas into the sink, pour the juices into the bowl of a stand mixer. Add ⅛ teaspoon cream of tartar and 2 tablespoons Swerve confectioners' sweetener and whip until stiff peaks form, about 10 minutes. Once peaks form, scoop it on top of your brownies and enjoy!

Ginger Triple Berry Crisp

Using three types of berries really makes the flavors in this crisp pop, but you can stick to one kind if you prefer. When you're ready to eat, you can eat this crisp cold or heat it up for about 30 seconds in the microwave and top it with some TruWhip for a real treat.

SERVES 6

Per Serving:

Calories	300
Fat	9g
Sodium	9mg
Carbohydrates	49g
Fiber	9g
Sugar	6g
Protein	6g

1 cup fresh blueberries
1 cup fresh blackberries
1 cup fresh raspberries
½ cup Swerve granular sweetener
1½ cups gluten-free rolled oats
½ cup Swerve brown sweetener
1 teaspoon ground cinnamon
½ teaspoon ground nutmeg
¼ teaspoon ground ginger
3 tablespoons unsalted grass-fed butter

1. Preheat oven to 350°F.
2. Combine berries and granular sweetener in a large bowl. Let sit 10 minutes.
3. In a separate large bowl, combine oats, brown sweetener, cinnamon, nutmeg, and ginger. Cut in butter until mixture gets crumbly.
4. Transfer berry mixture to an ungreased 9" × 9" baking dish and top with oat mixture. Bake 30 minutes or until topping starts to turn golden brown and crisp is bubbly. Remove from oven and allow to cool 1 hour.
5. Divide evenly into six airtight containers. Store in refrigerator until ready to eat, up to 1 week.

Two-Week Meal Plan

Week 1					
	Breakfast	Lunch	Snack	Dinner	Dessert
MON	Cinnamon Roll Overnight Oats	Barbecue Ranch Chicken Salad	Air-Fried Buffalo Cauliflower	Deconstructed Gyro Bowls	Double Chocolate Fudge Bites
TUE	Cinnamon Roll Overnight Oats	Barbecue Ranch Chicken Salad	Air-Fried Buffalo Cauliflower	Deconstructed Gyro Bowls	Double Chocolate Fudge Bites
WED	Spaghetti Squash Breakfast Bake	Barbecue Ranch Chicken Salad	Chocolate Chip Pumpkin Protein Muffins	Deconstructed Gyro Bowls	Edible Protein Cookie Dough
THU	Spaghetti Squash Breakfast Bake	Quinoa and Black Bean Power Bowls	Chocolate Chip Pumpkin Protein Muffins	Turkey-Stuffed Peppers	Edible Protein Cookie Dough
FRI	Spaghetti Squash Breakfast Bake	Quinoa and Black Bean Power Bowls	Chocolate Chip Pumpkin Protein Muffins	Turkey-Stuffed Peppers	Edible Protein Cookie Dough
SAT	Spaghetti Squash Breakfast Bake	Quinoa and Black Bean Power Bowls	Chocolate Chip Pumpkin Protein Muffins	Turkey-Stuffed Peppers	Edible Protein Cookie Dough
SUN	High-Protein Greek Yogurt Parfaits	Low-Carb Patty Melts	Sweet Potato and Zucchini Fritters	Baked Taquitos	Paleo Apple Pie Bars

Week 2					
	Breakfast	Lunch	Snack	Dinner	Dessert
MON	Chocolate Peanut Butter Chia Pudding Cups	Zoodle Pasta Salad	Maple Peanut Butter Oat Bars	Salsa Chicken	Strawberries with Chocolate Cheesecake Dip
TUE	Chocolate Peanut Butter Chia Pudding Cups	Zoodle Pasta Salad	Maple Peanut Butter Oat Bars	Salsa Chicken	Strawberries with Chocolate Cheesecake Dip
WED	Chocolate Peanut Butter Chia Pudding Cups	Zoodle Pasta Salad	Maple Peanut Butter Oat Bars	Salsa Chicken	Strawberries with Chocolate Cheesecake Dip
THU	Spaghetti Squash Breakfast Bake	Quinoa and Black Bean Power Bowls	Chocolate Chip Pumpkin Protein Muffins	Turkey-Stuffed Peppers	Edible Protein Cookie Dough
FRI	Spaghetti Squash Breakfast Bake	Quinoa and Black Bean Power Bowls	Chocolate Chip Pumpkin Protein Muffins	Turkey-Stuffed Peppers	Edible Protein Cookie Dough
SAT	Spaghetti Squash Breakfast Bake	Quinoa and Black Bean Power Bowls	Chocolate Chip Pumpkin Protein Muffins	Turkey-Stuffed Peppers	Edible Protein Cookie Dough
SUN	High-Protein Greek Yogurt Parfaits	Low-Carb Patty Melts	Sweet Potato and Zucchini Fritters	Baked Taquitos	Paleo Apple Pie Bars

STANDARD US/METRIC MEASUREMENT CONVERSIONS

VOLUME CONVERSIONS

US Volume Measure	Metric Equivalent
⅛ teaspoon	0.5 milliliter
¼ teaspoon	1 milliliter
½ teaspoon	2 milliliters
1 teaspoon	5 milliliters
½ tablespoon	7 milliliters
1 tablespoon (3 teaspoons)	15 milliliters
2 tablespoons (1 fluid ounce)	30 milliliters
¼ cup (4 tablespoons)	60 milliliters
⅓ cup	90 milliliters
½ cup (4 fluid ounces)	125 milliliters
⅔ cup	160 milliliters
¾ cup (6 fluid ounces)	180 milliliters
1 cup (16 tablespoons)	250 milliliters
1 pint (2 cups)	500 milliliters
1 quart (4 cups)	1 liter (about)

WEIGHT CONVERSIONS

US Weight Measure	Metric Equivalent
½ ounce	15 grams
1 ounce	30 grams
2 ounces	60 grams
3 ounces	85 grams
¼ pound (4 ounces)	115 grams
½ pound (8 ounces)	225 grams
¾ pound (12 ounces)	340 grams
1 pound (16 ounces)	454 grams

OVEN TEMPERATURE CONVERSIONS

Degrees Fahrenheit	Degrees Celsius
200 degrees F	95 degrees C
250 degrees F	120 degrees C
275 degrees F	135 degrees C
300 degrees F	150 degrees C
325 degrees F	160 degrees C
350 degrees F	180 degrees C
375 degrees F	190 degrees C
400 degrees F	205 degrees C
425 degrees F	220 degrees C
450 degrees F	230 degrees C

BAKING PAN SIZES

American	Metric
8 × 1½ inch round baking pan	20 × 4 cm cake tin
9 × 1½ inch round baking pan	23 × 3.5 cm cake tin
11 × 7 × 1½ inch baking pan	28 × 18 × 4 cm baking tin
13 × 9 × 2 inch baking pan	30 × 20 × 5 cm baking tin
2 quart rectangular baking dish	30 × 20 × 3 cm baking tin
15 × 10 × 2 inch baking pan	30 × 25 × 2 cm baking tin (Swiss roll tin)
9 inch pie plate	22 × 4 or 23 × 4 cm pie plate
7 or 8 inch springform pan	18 or 20 cm springform or loose bottom cake tin
9 × 5 × 3 inch loaf pan	23 × 13 × 7 cm or 2 lb narrow loaf or pate tin
1½ quart casserole	1.5 liter casserole
2 quart casserole	2 liter casserole

Index

Note: Page numbers in **bold** indicate recipe category lists.